I0838996

CONQUERING THE KIDNEY DIET

Thriving with CKD Through Nutrition

James Fabin

Dadvice TV - Kidney Health Coach

Copyright © 2023 James Fabin

All rights reserved

No part of this book may be reproduced, or stored in a retrieval system, or transmitted in any form or by any means, electronic, mechanical, photocopying, recording, or otherwise, without express written permission of the publisher.

Paperback ISBN: 9798851188695

Cover design by: James Fabin

Second Edition: August 2023

Limit of Liability/Disclaimer of Medical Advice

While the publisher and author have used their best efforts in writing and preparing this book, no representation or warranties exist with respect to the accuracy and completeness of this book, or that the contents apply to your current health or form of disease. The advice, research, diet, and plan may not be appropriate for all patients. A medical doctor should always assist you in making any treatment decisions, and patients should always be under the care and supervision of a physician. You should never make treatment decisions on your own without consulting a physician. Neither the author nor the publisher are liable for any medical decisions made based on the contents of this book. This includes special, incidental, consequential, or any other kinds of damages or liability.

Patients should always be under the care of a physician and defer to their physician for any and all treatment decisions. This book is not meant to replace a physician's advice, supervision, and counsel. No information in this book should be construed as medical advice. All medical decisions should be made by the patient and a qualified physician. This book is for informational purposes only.

To the unsung heroes of kidney health, the renal dietitians. This book is dedicated to you. With heartfelt admiration and gratitude, we honor your tireless devotion in guiding and supporting those battling kidney disease. You are the champions of nutrition, transforming lives and empowering patients to slow the progression of this relentless disease.

CONTENTS

INTRODUCTION

Welcome to "Conquering The Kidney Diet: Thriving with CKD Through Nutrition." If you are reading this, you or someone you care about is likely on a journey with kidney disease. I understand the challenges, fears, and uncertainties that come with this condition, as I have traversed this path myself. My personal experience inspired me to write my first book, "Conquering Kidney Disease: A survivor's guide to thriving with CKD," where I shared my story and provided a comprehensive understanding of Chronic Kidney Disease.

In this second book, we delve deeper into a crucial aspect of managing kidney disease: nutrition. The power of healthy food choices to reduce the burden placed on our kidneys cannot be underestimated. However, I want to make it clear from the start that this book is not a collection of recipes. Instead, it serves as a comprehensive guide to understanding the key elements of nutrition and their impact on kidney disease.

This book is not intended for those already on dialysis, but rather for individuals who are looking to manage their kidney disease, delay its progression, and potentially avoid the need for dialysis in the future. It is a guide to empower you with knowledge and practical strategies to make kidney-friendly food choices that support your well-being and longevity.

One of the greatest challenges for individuals newly diagnosed with kidney disease is the fear of food. Suddenly, the plate before them feels like a minefield of potential harm, and every bite carries the weight of uncertainty. But fear not, for this book aims to conquer that fear and empower you to embrace food again.

Through a deep exploration of the principles of the kidney diet, we will demystify the complexities and provide you with practical tools and insights. This book is designed to give you a solid foundation of knowledge so that you can make informed choices about the foods you eat. You will gain an understanding of the nutrients that support kidney health, learn to navigate food labels, and discover strategies for dining out and attending social events without fear.

By the end of this book, my hope is that you will feel empowered to enjoy food once more. You will be equipped with the knowledge and understanding to make kidney-friendly choices that not only nourish your body but also bring joy to your dining experience. No longer will you be paralyzed by anxiety or consumed by restrictive diets. Instead, you will embrace a balanced approach to nutrition, savoring the flavors and textures that make eating a pleasure.

Through the pages ahead, we will tackle the common misconceptions surrounding the kidney diet and provide evidence-based insights into the role of nutrition in managing kidney disease. We will explore the significance of portion control, discuss the impact of various nutrients on kidney health, and provide practical tips for incorporating healthy choices into your daily life.

So, let us embark on this transformative journey together. By understanding the key elements of nutrition and their impact on kidney disease, we can conquer the fear of food and reclaim our enjoyment of eating. This book will serve as your guide, your companion, and your source of knowledge and empowerment. Prepare to dine out without fear, attend events without worry, and experience the joy of nourishing your body in a way that supports your kidney health.

With warmest wishes for your well-being,

James Fabin

Dadvice TV Kidney Health Coach

THE KEY INGREDIENT: HOW I FOUND THE SECRET TO THRIVING WITH KIDNEY DISEASE

My CKD journey began with an unexpected twist that turned my life upside down. Little did I know that my kidneys were silently suffering, without any symptoms or warning signs. My story starts a year before my diagnosis, on a seemingly ordinary day. I was taking my kids and their grandpa out for ice cream when suddenly, a reckless driver failed to stop at an intersection and crashed into my SUV. The impact was so strong that it activated many of the airbags, including the side impact airbag built into my seat. The force of the airbags and the vehicle hitting the drive-side door pushed me against the center console, causing a lasting injury to my back. The force of the large vehicle slamming into my SUV caused my vehicle to spin in the intersection before coming to a halt, facing the opposite direction. My kid's grandpa was able to exit from the passenger side and help my kids and niece exit the vehicle. I was the last to be removed due to excruciating back pain and difficulty opening my crushed door, which marked the beginning of a long and arduous road to recovery.

I underwent therapy over the following 12 months to correct my spinal alignment, but the pain persisted. Lifting my small children, and common items, or sitting for too long became excruciating. It was sometimes painful to push a shopping cart, making routine tasks like getting groceries difficult. To cope with the back pain from my injuries, I relied on daily doses of Ibuprofen, always careful not to exceed the recommended dosage. At night I occasionally used Advil PM (ibuprofen with a sleeping agent) to help me sleep through the night while managing the back pain. Visits to a chiropractor were extremely helpful, and I reduced my reliance on Ibuprofen slowly, but I never went more than a few days without using it.

One fateful evening, 11.5 months after the accident, I started to feel unwell while enjoying famous Cincinnati chili dogs with my family to celebrate moving into our new home. As the night wore on, my condition rapidly deteriorated. I felt increasingly worse, reminiscent of a past bout of food poisoning just days before my wedding. Over the next two weeks, my body betrayed me, unleashing a cascade of debilitating symptoms. My vision blurred, a persistent cough wracked my chest, and I suffered from throbbing headaches, teeth-rattling chills, itchy skin, and uncontrollable diarrhea. The simple act of eating became a torment, as constant vomiting wracked my weakened body. My energy dwindled, and I struggled to focus through the haze of an unrelenting headache. It felt as if death itself was knocking at my door, the result of a merciless battle taking its toll on my very essence.

Unable to keep anything down, I would vomit everything I tried to consume, even my life-sustaining blood pressure medication. I survived on sports drinks and crackers for days, which were difficult to keep down. The consequences were dire. My blood pressure skyrocketed dangerously, and I teetered on the precipice of a life-threatening condition. Desperation and fear consumed me as I visited my family doctor, hoping for relief. I was confident it was food poisoning, which also inflamed my back pain. I explained that I couldn't take my blood pressure medication, which appeared to be why my blood pressure was so high. My family doctor gave me some medicine and a shot for the pain with instructions to return in 3 days for a follow-up.

Things were even worse the following day, and I knew I couldn't wait for the follow-up appointment. I had errands to complete as my family and I focused on unpacking and settling into our new home. I drove to my family doctor and used my dwindling strength to walk into the clinic, hopeful that a different medication would end my suffering. To my dismay, the severity of my condition was immediately apparent to him. He wasted no time and insisted I head straight to the emergency room. Although I initially hesitated, clinging to the idea of completing my errands, his stern warning left me no choice: if I didn't go immediately, he would call an ambulance to take me there. I was confronted with the reality that every moment mattered, that my life hung in the balance.

Arriving at the emergency room, I mustered the last remnants of my waning energy to exit my vehicle, only to collapse to the ground. The following moments, which stretched into hours, were a fight to stay conscious. I awoke in a wheelchair, my strength sapped by the relentless assault on my body and a lack of nourishment over the past two weeks. I remember being pushed through some doors, only to lose consciousness again. Then, as if in a haze, I found myself on a gurney, an IV needle piercing my arm. I continued to drift in and out of consciousness. Suddenly, I jolted awake; my arm, shoulder, and chest burned with an intensity that matched the inferno raging within, as the doctors administered potassium due to a blood test showing a critical deficiency. With treatment by the ER staff, I recovered enough to stay awake and answer questions. Finally, I was admitted to the Intensive Care Unit (ICU), which would become my new home for the next week.

While in the ICU, several doctors visited me, who looked at lab results, requested additional tests, and tried to figure out exactly what was wrong. My consistent cough continued, making it difficult to speak, sleep or hold still for an ultrasound. This was extremely confusing, and doctors would talk to me using medical terms I didn't understand. I recall hearing "Renal" repeatedly, and doctors continued to do blood tests and review the results. I had my wife bring me my iPad and laptop so I could do my own research. My focus was still on food poisoning; I was sure I could find something to help the doctors cure me faster.

On the second day in the ICU, a Nephrologist walked me through all the tests and their results – most of which I didn't understand. The phrase "renal failure" was repeated multiple times, but I had no clue what a "renal" was or what renal failure meant. I was still certain I was suffering from food poisoning, and the Nephrologist continued to try and convince me it wasn't. After the Nephrologist left, I researched online and learned about kidneys and kidney disease.

As I read more and more about kidney disease on the Internet, I became even more confused. As everyone who has looked up kidney disease online knows, there is a wealth of conflicting, scary, and even inaccurate information. I was able to make a list of questions to ask the Nephrologist (which I now understood what a Nephrologist was). When she returned to check on me, we had a more informed and productive conversation about my condition and future. In the midst of the medical chaos, the truth revealed itself with staggering clarity: my kidneys had failed, their once vibrant and vital function reduced to a mere flicker. With an eGFR of 8, the gravity of my situation unfolded before my disbelieving eyes when the Nephrologist told me I'd be dead within 45 days without dialysis.

The initial shock and fear were overwhelming. Questions flooded my mind, each more haunting than the last: What did dialysis mean for my future? How would it impact my daily life, my dreams, my aspirations? Was there a cure, a glimmer of hope in the darkness? And the thought that haunted me most: Would I be able to go home, continue my work, and be there for my loved ones?

Determined to unravel the truth of my condition, I embarked on a relentless pursuit of knowledge. Hours were spent immersed in the depths of research, seeking answers and solace. I discovered that kidney disease was not a death sentence, that other countries with fewer resources than my own were achieving better outcomes in kidney care. Their success hinged on a holistic approach, addressing diet, lifestyle changes, and medications to manage blood pressure and symptoms. It became painfully clear that my country, the United States, lagged far behind in the quest for excellence in kidney care.

Despite the bleak prognosis delivered by my nephrologist, who insisted on dialysis, a glimmer of hope flickered deep within my soul. It was a hope nurtured by the research I had unearthed, by the stories of resilience and triumph that whispered in the dark corners of my mind. In that moment, I made a choice. I chose to fight kidney disease with every fiber of my being.

After 6 days in the ICU, my eGFR slightly improved, but it remained worryingly low. Dialysis loomed on the horizon, a formidable specter ready to claim me. However, I made a bold decision, fueled by a cocktail of hope and defiance. I refused to succumb to the fate prescribed by conventional wisdom. Instead, I embarked on a path less traveled, a path paved with dietary and lifestyle changes that promised a glimmer of salvation.

My journey to reclaim my health was not without its trials and tribulations. It required unwavering commitment, relentless discipline, and an unyielding spirit. With the guidance of my healthcare team, I discovered the perfect combination of blood pressure medications and implemented significant modifications to my diet. And as the days turned into weeks and the weeks into months, a miraculous transformation began to unfold. My eGFR climbed steadily, and with each passing day, my symptoms receded like shadows before the dawn. Energy surged through my veins, and I walked up to five miles a day, a testament to the indomitable spirit within.

I chronicled my experiences, battles, mistakes, and victories throughout this challenging odyssey. Like every person I've met with kidney disease, I searched for a quick fix or cure. I bombarded my doctors with questions about every kidney fix, flush, restore, or other solution I found online claiming to help with kidney disease. I fooled myself into believing there must be some special herb or supplement that would magically repair my kidneys and undue the scaring and damage. The number of fake fixes online only fueled my belief that there must be something to help that ever doctor on earth had overlooked. I eventually realized these were solutions pushed by evil people looking for a quick buck, taking advantage of our illness to fill their wallets. I discovered the real solution is through diet and lifestyle changes, all powered by a deeper understanding of kidney disease and our bodies. My health improved as I executed this new strategy, and the fears of needing dialysis faded into the background.

My story became a beacon of hope, a source of solace for others navigating the treacherous waters of kidney disease. It was through the sharing of my journey that Dadvice TV was born, a platform that brought together individuals with kidney disease, healthcare professionals, and researchers. Together, we became a community, a force of resilience, and a source of knowledge. Dadvice TV became a sanctuary of hope, compassion, and unwavering support.

Today, my website, DadviceTV.com, and my YouTube channel, Dadvice TV, serve as beacons of inspiration, reaching people across the globe. They provide a lifeline for those yearning for answers, for those desperate to regain control of their lives. My eGFR has stabilized in the low 30s, a testament to the power of determination and unwavering faith. I am now free from the shackles of debilitating symptoms, embracing life's myriad joys with unbridled enthusiasm. With my children, I explore new horizons, create cherished memories, and revel in the beauty of every precious moment.

By embarking on an extraordinary journey of self-discovery and empowerment, I have realized the profound impact my choices regarding lifestyle and the foods I consume have on my overall health and well-being. Through healthy living and nutrition, I have unlocked the key to my health improvement, transforming my body and revitalizing my spirit. Each mindful decision I make to nourish my body with wholesome, nutrient-rich foods serves as a powerful act of self-love, allowing me to reduce the stress and burden placed on my kidneys, and granting them the opportunity to perform their vital functions more effectively than ever before.

While my healthcare team has tirelessly worked to manage my blood pressure, anemia, and other symptoms, adopting a heart-healthy and kidney-friendly diet has propelled my journey towards remarkable improvement. By carefully selecting foods that nourish my body and support its optimal function, I have become an active participant in my treatment, amplifying the efficacy of medical interventions and accelerating my overall improvements.

Yet, let it be known that the road I tread is not without its challenges. The truth remains that my kidneys bear the scars of irreparable damage, and the realities of their limitations are ever-present. Nonetheless, armed with the profound understanding that my choices hold the power to shape my destiny, I remain resolute in my commitment to honor and nurture my body. Each day, I embrace the principles of a kidney-friendly diet, guided by the expert insights of a renal dietitian, who sets daily nutritional targets tailored to my unique needs. Armed with the invaluable assistance of a food-tracking app, I navigate the labyrinth of dietary choices with unwavering precision, ensuring that I remain steadfastly on the path to wellness. Moreover, I have embraced the transformative concept of portion control, recognizing that moderation is the key to safeguarding the delicate balance within.

As I traverse this journey, I know that my triumphs are

not defined solely by lab results and medical milestones. They transcend the physical realm, echoing in the resounding chorus of life's joys and the symphony of unforgettable moments. With profound gratitude, I acknowledge the immeasurable support of my healthcare team, whose tireless efforts have paved the way for my progress. They have served as steadfast guides, illuminating the path with their unwavering expertise and compassionate care.

Through sharing my personal story, I hope to ignite a flame of inspiration within the hearts of others who may find themselves facing a similar journey. I yearn to awaken their inner strength, encouraging them to seize control of their health and embrace the transformative power of nutrition and lifestyle choices. Together, we can embark upon a shared quest to navigate the labyrinth of kidney disease with unwavering courage and resilience. Bound by our collective determination, we find solace in knowing we are not alone on this arduous path. We are supported by the unwavering love of our cherished ones and the unyielding dedication of our healthcare professionals.

In the face of adversity, we possess an unconquerable spirit that defies the odds. We have the power to rewrite the narrative of our lives, embracing our newfound vitality and savoring the gift of each precious moment. Our unwavering commitment to nourishing our bodies allows us to breathe life into our wildest dreams and seize the boundless opportunities that lie before us. As we stand united in our journey of transformation, we become beacons of hope, casting light upon the path of others who yearn for a brighter future. Together, we embody the resounding truth that even amidst the shadows of adversity, we can rise above, not only to survive but to thrive in the realm of endless possibilities.

UNDERSTANDING KIDNEY DISEASE

OVERVIEW OF KIDNEY DISEASE AND ITS IMPACT ON OVERALL HEALTH

Kidney disease, also known as renal disease, is a complex condition that affects the functioning of the kidneys, essential organs responsible for filtering waste products, excess fluids, and toxins from the blood. These bean-shaped organs, located in the lower back, also play a crucial role in regulating blood pressure, electrolyte balance, and red blood cell production.

When kidney function becomes impaired or compromised, waste products, fluids, and electrolytes can build up in the body, leading to a range of symptoms and complications. The two main types of kidney disease are acute kidney injury (AKI), which occurs suddenly and often as a result of another underlying condition or medication, and chronic kidney disease (CKD), a progressive condition that develops over months or years.

CKD is typically characterized by five stages, ranging from mild kidney damage (Stage 1) to kidney failure, eventually requiring dialysis or transplantation (Stage 5 or end-stage renal disease, ESRD). Common causes of kidney disease include high blood pressure (hypertension), diabetes, autoimmune diseases, inherited disorders, urinary tract infections, kidney stones, and certain medications.

While there is currently no cure for kidney disease, adopting a healthy kidney diet and lifestyle can play a crucial role in managing the condition, alleviating symptoms, and slowing its progression. It is important to understand that a kidney-friendly diet, along with other recommended treatments and medications prescribed by healthcare professionals, can significantly improve your quality of life. However, it is essential to remain cautious and vigilant as there are individuals and companies who may prey on the vulnerability of those with kidney disease. Scam artists may attempt to sell fake cures, miracle fixes, and unproven treatments that claim to reverse or cure kidney disease. It is vital to rely on reputable sources of information, consult with your healthcare team, and be wary of any claims that seem too good to be true. Your health and well-being deserve evidence-based care and support, so always prioritize proven methods and treatments backed by scientific research and medical expertise.

IMPORTANCE OF NUTRITION IN MANAGING KIDNEY DISEASE

Nutrition plays a pivotal role in managing kidney disease and optimizing overall health for individuals with compromised kidney function. A kidney-friendly diet is designed to reduce the workload on the kidneys, minimize the accumulation of waste products, control blood pressure, manage fluid and electrolyte balance, and preserve kidney function for as long as possible.

Proper nutrition is vital in the management of kidney disease for several reasons:

Minimizing Kidney Stress: By carefully selecting and controlling nutrient intake, individuals with kidney disease can reduce the strain on their kidneys. Limiting the consumption of certain nutrients helps prevent the buildup of waste products that healthy kidneys would usually filter and excrete.

Blood Pressure Control: High blood pressure is a common complication of kidney disease and can further damage the kidneys. Following a kidney-friendly diet, which emphasizes whole foods, reduces sodium intake, and promotes a balanced intake of other key nutrients, can help maintain healthy blood pressure levels.

Fluid and Electrolyte Balance: The kidneys play a crucial role in maintaining fluid and electrolyte balance in the body. For individuals with kidney disease, maintaining the appropriate fluid balance is essential to prevent fluid retention and manage conditions such as edema or swelling. Controlling electrolyte levels, such as potassium and phosphorus, is also crucial to avoid imbalances that can lead to complications.

Preserving Kidney Function: A well-managed diet can help slow the progression of kidney disease, extending the period during which individuals can maintain kidney function without relying on dialysis or transplantation. It can also help manage complications and improve overall quality of life.

THE ROLE OF DIET IN SUPPORTING KIDNEY HEALTH

Diet plays a significant role in supporting kidney health and managing kidney disease. A kidney-friendly diet focuses on optimizing nutrient intake while controlling the intake of specific nutrients that can burden the kidneys or contribute to complications.

Here are key principles of a kidney-friendly diet:

- Sodium Management
- Phosphorus Control
- Protein Moderation
- Potassium Regulation
- Fluid Control

In addition to these key principles, a kidney-friendly diet emphasizes the importance of consuming a variety of nutrient-dense foods. This includes incorporating fruits, vegetables, whole grains, and healthy fats into your meals while being mindful of portion sizes and cooking methods that minimize the use of added fats, sugars, and excessive salt.

By adopting a kidney-friendly diet, individuals with kidney disease can support their kidney health, manage complications, and slow the progression of the disease. However, it is important to note that dietary recommendations **may vary** depending on the stage of kidney disease, individual needs, and other underlying health conditions. Working closely with a registered dietitian who specializes in renal nutrition can provide personalized guidance and support in developing a tailored nutrition plan.

In the chapters that follow, we will delve deeper into specific nutrients, explore strategies for meal planning and preparation, discuss dietary considerations for dining out and special occasions, address common questions and concerns, and provide a variety of kidney-friendly recipes. By understanding kidney disease and the role of nutrition, you will be empowered to take control of your health and make informed choices that promote optimal kidney function and overall well-being. Let's embark on this journey together towards a healthier, thriving life with kidney disease.

ONE SIZE DOESN'T FIT ALL

It is crucial to emphasize that kidney disease is a complex condition with unique variations and individualized needs. There is no "one size fits all" diet that can be applied universally to everyone with kidney disease. Each person's nutritional requirements must be personalized and tailored to their specific health status, underlying conditions, lab results, lifestyle, and activity level.

For instance, even individuals with the same level of kidney function may have different dietary needs. While one person may require a potassium restriction due to their specific health conditions or lab results, another person with similar kidney function may need to increase their potassium intake to address deficiencies or other health concerns. This highlights the importance of **individualizing the diet** according to the unique needs of each person.

Determining the appropriate nutritional approach involves considering factors beyond kidney function. Health conditions such as diabetes, high blood pressure, and heart disease, as well as individual factors like age, weight, medications, and dietary preferences, must be taken into account. Regular monitoring of lab results and close collaboration with healthcare professionals and registered dietitians who specialize in renal nutrition are crucial in developing a personalized dietary plan.

By recognizing that the level of kidney function alone does not dictate the diet, we empower individuals with kidney disease to take an active role in their own health. By working with healthcare professionals to assess their specific needs, individuals can develop a diet that optimally supports their kidney health while addressing their unique nutritional requirements.

UNRAVELING THE KIDNEY-HEALTHY DIET PUZZLE

In this chapter, we will explore the intricate details of a kidney-healthy diet, focusing on the key principles that form its foundation. By understanding these principles, you will gain a comprehensive understanding of how to nourish your kidneys and support your overall well-being. We will delve into guidelines for managing essential nutrients such as sodium, phosphorus, protein, potassium, and fluid intake. Additionally, we will discuss the art of balancing nutrition and taste to achieve optimal results without compromising on flavor.

KEY PRINCIPLES OF A KIDNEY-FRIENDLY DIET

A kidney-friendly diet revolves around specific principles that promote kidney health and help manage the progression of kidney disease. By incorporating these principles into your dietary choices, you can optimize your well-being. Let's delve a little deeper into the key principles:

Sodium Management: High sodium levels can contribute to fluid retention and increased blood pressure, putting strain on the kidneys. To manage sodium intake, it is crucial to limit the consumption of processed and packaged foods, which are typically high in sodium. Instead, opt for fresh, whole foods prepared with herbs, spices, and other sodium-free seasonings to enhance the flavor of your meals. By embracing these changes, you can maintain healthy blood pressure and minimize fluid retention.

Phosphorus Control: The kidneys play a vital role in regulating phosphorus levels in the body. In kidney disease, impaired kidney function can lead to difficulties in filtering and excreting phosphorus, which can contribute to bone and cardiovascular complications. To manage phosphorus intake, it is essential to limit the consumption of high-phosphorus foods such as dairy products, processed meats, carbonated beverages, and certain processed foods. By working closely with your healthcare team or registered dietitian, you can develop a personalized plan that ensures appropriate phosphorus control.

Protein Moderation: Protein is an essential nutrient for maintaining overall health. However, excessive protein intake can place a burden on the kidneys. In kidney disease, it is important to moderate protein consumption to reduce the production of waste products that the kidneys must filter. High-quality protein sources, such as lean meats, poultry, fish, eggs, and plant-based proteins like legumes and tofu, should be selected. By monitoring portion sizes and working with your healthcare team or registered dietitian, you can determine the appropriate protein intake for your individual needs.

Potassium Regulation: Potassium is a mineral necessary for various bodily functions, including maintaining normal heart rhythm and muscle function. In kidney disease, imbalances in potassium levels can be detrimental to health. It is important to manage potassium intake based on individual circumstances. Depending on your specific needs, you may need to limit or increase potassium consumption. High-potassium foods, such as bananas, oranges, tomatoes, potatoes, and avocadoes, may need to be restricted or incorporated into your diet in moderation. Working closely with your healthcare team or registered dietitian will help you develop a personalized plan that ensures optimal potassium regulation.

Fluid Management: Proper fluid management is essential for individuals with kidney disease to maintain hydration and prevent fluid overload. Fluid restrictions may be necessary, depending on various factors such as urine output, stage of kidney disease, and other medical conditions. Working closely with your healthcare team or registered dietitian will help you determine the appropriate fluid intake for your individual needs. By monitoring your fluid intake and being mindful of thirst cues, you can effectively manage fluid balance and support kidney health.

GUIDELINES FOR MANAGING SODIUM, PHOSPHORUS, PROTEIN, POTASSIUM, AND FLUID INTAKE

To effectively manage essential nutrients, it is important to have a clear understanding of the guidelines for each. Here are some general guidelines to consider:

Sodium Management: Limiting sodium intake to recommended levels, typically 1500 to 2300 milligrams per day, is crucial for individuals with kidney disease. This involves minimizing the use of table salt and reducing consumption of processed and packaged foods, which are often high in sodium. Instead, focus on fresh, whole foods prepared with herbs, spices, and other sodium-free seasonings to enhance flavor while keeping sodium levels in check.

Phosphorus Control: Controlling phosphorus intake is essential in managing kidney disease. It is generally recommended to limit phosphorus consumption to approximately 800 to 1200 milligrams per day. This involves avoiding high-phosphorus foods such as dairy products, processed meats, carbonated beverages, and certain processed foods. It may also be necessary to take phosphorus binders with meals to help limit phosphorus absorption. Working closely with your healthcare team or registered dietitian will ensure an individualized approach that meets your specific phosphorus needs.

Protein Moderation: Moderating protein intake is important to lessen the strain on the kidneys. The recommended protein intake varies depending on individual factors such as stage of kidney disease, nutritional status, and other health conditions. Generally, a range of 0.6 to 0.8 gram of protein per kilogram of body weight per day is advised for individuals with kidney disease who are not on dialysis. However, individual needs may differ, and consulting with your healthcare team or registered dietitian will help determine the appropriate protein intake for you.

Potassium Regulation: Balancing potassium levels is crucial, and the specific recommendations for potassium intake depend on your individual circumstances. While some individuals with kidney disease may need to limit potassium intake, others may require increased potassium consumption. High-potassium foods such as bananas, oranges, tomatoes, potatoes, and avocadoes may need to be restricted or incorporated into the diet in moderation. Working closely with your healthcare team or registered dietitian will ensure that your potassium intake aligns with your specific needs.

Fluid Management: Effective fluid management is essential for maintaining proper hydration and preventing fluid overload. The recommended fluid intake varies based on individual factors such as urine output, stage of kidney disease, and other medical conditions. Following the guidance of your healthcare team or registered dietitian will help determine the appropriate fluid restriction or allowance for you. Monitoring your fluid intake and being mindful of thirst cues can aid in maintaining a healthy fluid balance.

QUESTIONS TO ASK YOUR HEALTHCARE TEAM

To ensure that your kidney-friendly diet is personalized and aligned with your specific needs, it is essential to have open and informative discussions with your healthcare team or dietitian. Here are some important questions to ask them:

How many calories do I need?

Understanding your daily caloric needs is crucial for maintaining a healthy weight and overall well-being. Your healthcare team can provide guidance on the appropriate calorie intake based on factors such as your age, sex, weight, activity level, and specific health conditions.

Do I need to limit how much protein I eat? If so, how many grams of protein should I consume per day?

Protein intake needs to be managed in kidney disease to reduce the workload on the kidneys. Your healthcare team can help determine the appropriate amount of protein for your individual needs, considering factors such as the stage of your kidney disease and your nutritional status.

What does a balanced meal include? What are good snacks?

Understanding the components of a balanced meal is essential for meeting your nutritional needs while managing kidney disease. Your healthcare team can provide guidance on including appropriate amounts of protein, carbohydrates, healthy fats, and essential nutrients in your meals. They can also suggest suitable kidney-friendly snacks that align with your dietary restrictions.

Is my potassium level too high or low? How much potassium should I target each day?

Managing potassium levels is crucial in kidney disease, as imbalances can affect heart health. Your healthcare team can assess your potassium levels and recommend a target range for daily potassium intake. They can also provide information about high-potassium and low-potassium food choices to help you achieve the right balance.

Is my phosphorus level too high? Should I restrict my phosphorus intake?

Phosphorus management is important in kidney disease to prevent complications such as bone and cardiovascular problems. Your healthcare team can evaluate your phosphorus levels and advise you on whether you need to restrict phosphorus in your diet. They can also guide you on selecting low-phosphorus food options and provide strategies for phosphorus control.

How much sodium (salt) should I consume?

Reducing sodium intake is crucial for managing blood pressure and fluid balance in kidney disease. Your healthcare team can provide specific recommendations for your sodium intake based on your health status and goals. They can also offer strategies for reducing sodium in your diet and suggest alternative ways to enhance flavor without relying on excessive salt.

How many ounces of fluid are right for me?

Managing fluid intake is essential for individuals with kidney disease, especially those with fluid retention or compromised kidney function. Your healthcare team can assess your fluid needs and provide personalized recommendations on how much fluid you should consume daily. They can also help you develop strategies to monitor and manage fluid intake effectively.

Do I need a nutritional supplement? If so, which one is right for me?

Supplements may be necessary in some cases to address specific nutritional deficiencies or meet increased nutrient needs. Your healthcare team can evaluate your nutritional status and advise you on whether you need a nutritional supplement. They can recommend appropriate supplements based on your individual requirements.

Should I take vitamins?

Vitamin requirements may vary in kidney disease, and supplementation may be necessary in certain situations. Your healthcare team can assess your vitamin levels and provide recommendations on whether you should take specific vitamins. They can guide you on the appropriate dosage and help you choose high-quality supplements if needed.

What strategies can help slow the progression of my CKD?

Slowing the progression of CKD is an essential goal in its management. Your healthcare team can provide valuable insights and strategies to help protect your kidney function.

This may include recommendations on dietary modifications, lifestyle changes, medication management, and regular monitoring to optimize kidney health.

BALANCING NUTRITION AND TASTE FOR OPTIMAL RESULTS

Achieving optimal results in a kidney-healthy diet does not mean compromising on taste. By implementing strategies to balance nutrition and flavor, you can create delicious and satisfying meals. Consider the following:

Embrace Herbs and Spices: Incorporating a wide variety of herbs, spices, and seasonings into your cooking can add depth and flavor to your meals without relying on excessive salt or sodium. Experiment with different combinations to discover exciting flavors that enhance your dishes.

Explore Cooking Techniques: Adopt cooking methods such as grilling, baking, steaming, or stir-frying to bring out the natural flavors of foods while minimizing the need for added fats or salt. These techniques help retain nutrients and create enjoyable dishes.

Modify Recipes: Adapt recipes to fit your kidney-healthy diet. Substitute ingredients, adjust portion sizes, and modify cooking methods to meet your nutritional needs while maintaining delicious flavors. Get creative and experiment with new combinations and cooking styles.

Personalize to Your Preferences: Take your personal taste preferences into account when planning meals. Tailor recipes to suit your likes and dislikes, making sure that the kidney-healthy diet remains enjoyable and sustainable for you.

Remember, a kidney-healthy diet is not a one-size-fits-all approach. Individualizing the diet based on your specific needs, recommendations from your healthcare team or registered dietitian, and close monitoring of your progress and lab results is crucial. Working closely with your healthcare team or registered dietitian will ensure that your dietary plan is tailored to your unique health profile and goals.

By adhering to the key principles of a kidney-friendly diet, you can support your kidney health, manage complications, and enhance your overall well-being. The guidelines for managing sodium, phosphorus, protein, potassium, and fluid intake provide a framework for making informed choices. However, it is important to emphasize that these guidelines are not universal and may vary based on your individual circumstances.

The art of balancing nutrition and taste is an ongoing process that allows you to create flavorful meals while meeting your nutritional needs. Embracing herbs, spices, and cooking techniques can elevate the taste of your dishes without relying on excessive salt or sodium. Modifying recipes and personalizing them to your preferences ensures that you find joy and satisfaction in your kidney-healthy diet.

Remember, you are the driver of your own health journey. By working closely with your healthcare team, registered dietitian, and incorporating these principles into your daily life, you can navigate the complexities of a kidney-healthy diet with confidence. Your commitment to optimal nutrition will contribute to the well-being of your kidneys and overall health.

PORTION CONTROL: THE SECRET TO SUCCESS

Portion control plays a vital role in managing kidney disease and maintaining overall health. By understanding the significance of portion control, you can enjoy your meals without the fear of causing harm to your kidneys. In this chapter, we will delve into the details of portion control, including its significance, recommended serving sizes for different food groups, practical tips for practicing portion control at home and when dining out, and strategies for maintaining portion control as a long-term habit.

UNDERSTANDING THE SIGNIFICANCE OF PORTION CONTROL IN MANAGING KIDNEY DISEASE

Portion control is a game-changer when it comes to managing kidney disease. It not only helps you regulate nutrient intake and maintain a healthy weight but also transforms how you view a kidney-friendly diet. Rather than focusing on a long list of foods you cannot eat, portion control empowers you to enjoy a wide variety of foods, as long as you practice moderation.

For individuals with kidney disease, it's important to be

mindful of certain nutrients such as sugar, sodium, and phosphorus. Portion control allows you to indulge in these foods in smaller quantities, allowing for a more flexible and satisfying eating experience. This shift in mindset alleviates the fear and anxiety that often accompanies a restricted diet, as you realize that you can still enjoy your favorite foods as long as you do not overdo it.

One common challenge for newly diagnosed kidney patients is the fear of food. The overwhelming desire to avoid potential harm can lead to over-restriction, which can result in inadequate nutrient intake and even malnutrition. However, with portion control, this fear is replaced with a sense of empowerment. You can approach your meals with confidence, knowing that you can savor the flavors and textures you love while still prioritizing your kidney health.

By understanding portion control, you gain a newfound sense of control over your diet. Instead of feeling deprived or restricted, you have the freedom to make choices that align with your health goals. You become an active participant in your journey towards improved kidney health, no longer held back by fear or confusion.

Implementing portion control does not mean you have to measure every morsel of food you eat. It is about developing a sense of awareness and intuitively gauging appropriate portion sizes. This can be achieved through visual cues, such as using your hand as a guide for portion estimation or observing the proportions of different food groups on your plate.

Through portion control, you can still enjoy your favorite dishes and maintain a well-balanced diet. By including a variety of fruits, vegetables, whole grains, lean proteins, and low-fat dairy products in appropriate portions, you can meet your nutritional needs while managing kidney disease.

EXPLORING PORTION SIZES AND RECOMMENDED SERVINGS FOR DIFFERENT FOOD GROUPS

Understanding portion sizes and recommended servings for different food groups is crucial for practicing portion control and maintaining a balanced diet. Here are some general guidelines to help you navigate portion sizes for various food groups:

1. Non-Starchy Vegetables:
   a. Recommended Servings: Aim for 2 to 3 servings per meal.
   b. Portion Size Examples: 1 cup raw leafy greens, 1/2 cup cooked vegetables, 1/2 cup vegetable juice.
2. Starchy Vegetables and Grains:
   a. Recommended Servings: Limit starchy vegetables and grains to 1 to 2 servings per meal.
   b. Portion Size Examples: 1/2 cup cooked rice, pasta, or grains; 1 small potato or sweet potato; 1 slice of bread.
3. Protein Sources:
   a. Recommended Servings: Consume 3 to 4 ounces (about the size of a deck of cards) of protein per meal.
   b. Portion Size Examples: 3 to 4 ounces of lean meat, poultry, or fish; 1/2 cup cooked beans or legumes; 2 to 3 eggs; 1 ounce of cheese.

4. Dairy or Dairy Alternatives:

   a. Recommended Servings: Aim for 1 to 2 servings per meal.

   b. Portion Size Examples: 1 cup of milk or yogurt, 1.5 ounces of cheese, or a calcium-fortified dairy alternative.

5. Fruits:

   a. Recommended Servings: Include 1 to 2 servings of fruits per meal.

   b. Portion Size Examples: 1 medium-sized fruit (such as an apple or orange), 1/2 cup of chopped fruit, or 1/4 cup of dried fruit.

6. Fats and Oils:

   a. Recommended Servings: Use fats and oils sparingly.

   b. Portion Size Examples: 1 teaspoon of oil, 1 tablespoon of nut butter, or 1/8 of an avocado.

It's important to note that these portion sizes are general recommendations and may vary depending on individual needs, health conditions, and goals. Working with a renal dietitian can help provide more specific guidance tailored to your unique circumstances.

Keep in mind that portion control is not about strict deprivation but rather finding a balance that works for you. Adjust portion sizes based on your hunger levels, activity levels, and overall health goals. Be mindful of the total calorie content of your meals and consider incorporating a variety of foods from different food groups to ensure you receive a diverse range of nutrients.

When portioning your meals, it can be helpful to use visual cues and everyday objects as references. For example, a 3-ounce serving of meat is roughly the size of a deck of cards, while 1 cup of cooked grains is similar in size to a tennis ball. Experiment with different portion control tools, such as measuring cups and food scales, until you become more familiar with appropriate serving sizes.

TIPS FOR PRACTICING PORTION CONTROL AT HOME AND WHEN DINING OUT

Practicing portion control is essential for managing kidney disease, both at home and when dining out. It helps you maintain a balanced diet, control calorie intake, and ensure that you are not overloading your kidneys with excessive nutrients. Here are some practical tips to help you implement portion control in your everyday life:

Measure and Use Portion Control Tools: Use measuring cups, spoons, and a food scale to accurately measure your food portions. This will help you become familiar with appropriate serving sizes and ensure that you are not inadvertently consuming more than necessary.

Plate Method: The plate method is a visual guide that can help you create balanced and portion-controlled meals. Fill half of your plate with non-starchy vegetables like broccoli, spinach, or peppers. Use one-quarter of the plate for lean proteins such as grilled chicken, fish, or tofu. Reserve the remaining quarter for whole grains or starchy vegetables like brown rice, quinoa, or sweet potatoes.

Practice Mindful Eating: Slow down and pay attention to your body's hunger and fullness cues. Eat slowly, savoring each bite, and pause between bites to check if you are still hungry. By being more mindful, you can avoid overeating and better gauge when you are satisfied.

Use Smaller Plates and Bowls: Opt for smaller plates and bowls to visually trick your brain into thinking you have a full plate. This can help you feel satisfied with smaller portions. Avoid oversized plates, as they can lead to overeating and a distorted perception of serving sizes.

Pre-portion Snacks: Instead of eating snacks straight from the package, pre-portion them into smaller bags or containers. This prevents mindless eating and helps you control the amount you consume.

Fill Up on Fiber: Include fiber-rich foods like fruits, vegetables, whole grains, and legumes in your meals. These foods provide bulk and help you feel full for longer, reducing the temptation to overeat.

Be Mindful of Liquid Calories: Beverages can contribute significant calories to your diet. Be mindful of sugary drinks, fruit juices, and alcohol, as they can quickly add up. Opt for water, unsweetened tea, or other low-calorie options to quench your thirst.

When dining out, portion control can be more challenging due to larger serving sizes and limited control over ingredient choices. However, with these strategies, you can still enjoy a meal outside while managing your portions:

Share Meals: Consider splitting a meal with a dining companion or asking for a to-go box right away to portion out half of your meal before you start eating. This helps control portion sizes and prevents overeating.

Choose Smaller Portions: Look for menu options that offer smaller portion sizes or choose appetizers or side dishes instead of a full-sized entree. You can also ask for half-portions or children's sizes.

Request Sauces and Dressings on the Side: By requesting sauces, dressings, and condiments on the side, you have more control over the amount you use. Use them sparingly or opt for healthier alternatives like lemon juice or vinegar for added flavor.

Be Mindful of Sides: Restaurant meals often come with a variety of sides. Choose healthier options like steamed vegetables, side salads, or whole grains instead of fried or high-calorie choices.

Listen to Your Body: Pay attention to your body's signals of fullness and stop eating when you feel satisfied. Resist the urge to finish your plate just because it is there.

STRATEGIES FOR MAINTAINING PORTION CONTROL AS A LONG-TERM HABIT

Practicing portion control is not a temporary solution but a long-term lifestyle change that can support your kidney health and overall well-being. Here are some strategies to help you maintain portion control as a sustainable habit:

1. Plan and Prepare Meals:

   a. Take time to plan your meals in advance, considering portion sizes and incorporating a variety of food groups.

   b. Use portion control aids such as measuring cups, food scales, and portioned containers to help with meal preparation.

   c. Pre-portion snacks and meals into individual servings to avoid overeating.

2. Be Mindful of Hunger and Fullness Cues:

   a. Listen to your body's hunger and fullness cues. Eat slowly and pay attention to your level of satisfaction during meals.

   b. Stop eating when you feel comfortably satisfied, rather than overeating until you are overly full.

   c. Avoid distractions such as television or electronic devices while eating, as they can lead to mindless eating and larger portions.

3. Opt for Smaller Plates and Bowls:

   a. Use smaller plates and bowls to visually trick yourself into thinking you are consuming larger portions.

   b. This can help create a perception of a satisfying meal even with smaller portion sizes.

4. Fill Half Your Plate with Non-Starchy Vegetables:

   a. Non-starchy vegetables are low in calories and high in nutrients. Fill half your plate with non-starchy vegetables, such as leafy greens, broccoli, cauliflower, or peppers.

b. This helps to add bulk to your meal, making it more satisfying without significantly increasing calorie intake.

5. Be Mindful of Liquid Calories:

   a. Be cautious of liquid calories, such as sugary beverages or excessive amounts of fruit juice.

   b. Choose water or unsweetened beverages as your main hydration source, and limit high-calorie drinks that provide little nutritional value.

6. Practice Portion Control When Dining Out:

   a. When eating out, be mindful of larger portion sizes often served at restaurants.

   b. Consider sharing a meal with a friend or taking a portion of your meal home for later.

   c. Ask for dressings, sauces, and toppings on the side, allowing you to control the amount you consume.

7. Practice Self-Care and Manage Stress:

   a. Emotional eating and stress can lead to overeating and a lack of portion control.

   b. Find alternative ways to cope with stress, such as engaging in physical activity, practicing relaxation techniques, or seeking support from friends and family.

8. Keep a Food Journal:

   a. Keep a food journal to track your food intake, portion sizes, and feelings associated with eating.

    b. This can help create awareness around your eating habits, identify triggers for overeating, and hold yourself accountable.

9. Seek Support and Guidance:

    a. Work with a renal dietitian who can provide personalized guidance on portion control and help you navigate your specific dietary needs.

    b. Join support groups or online communities focused on kidney health, where you can connect with others facing similar challenges and share tips and strategies.

THE DADVICE TV KIDNEY DIET STRATEGY

The Dadvice TV Kidney Diet Strategy is a personalized approach to a kidney-friendly diet that prioritizes individual needs and empowers individuals to take control of their nutrition. This strategy encompasses several key elements that are essential for success in managing kidney disease, but it is not the only option. Let's explore the key elements and how they work.

INDIVIDUALIZATION WITH A RENAL DIETITIAN

Individualization with a Renal Dietitian is a cornerstone of the Dadvice TV Kidney Diet Strategy, underscoring the fact that food lists or common diets do not provide effective solutions for managing kidney disease. Even if two individuals have the same stage or level of kidney function, their dietary needs can vary significantly. It is essential to work with a renal dietitian to develop a personalized approach that suits your specific circumstances. This point is of utmost importance, and it will be reiterated throughout this book to emphasize its significance in achieving optimal kidney health.

Recognizing the Variability of Kidney Disease: Kidney

disease affects individuals in different ways, depending on factors such as the stage of the disease, underlying conditions, and overall health. What works for one person may not work for another, which is why a personalized approach is essential. A renal dietitian has the expertise to assess your unique situation and develop a diet plan that aligns with your specific needs, taking into account factors such as nutrient requirements, fluid restrictions, and potential interactions with medications. By individualizing your diet, you can address the specific challenges and goals you face in managing your kidney disease.

Tailoring Nutritional Recommendations: A renal dietitian will provide you with tailored nutritional recommendations based on your lab results, medical history, lifestyle, and personal preferences. They will help you understand the impact of different nutrients on your kidney health and guide you in making informed choices. For example, if you have high blood pressure or diabetes in addition to kidney disease, the dietitian will consider these factors when developing your dietary plan. They may provide guidelines on sodium intake, sugar control, and managing other comorbidities to support your overall health. By working closely with a renal dietitian, you can ensure that your diet is designed specifically for you, addressing your unique nutritional needs and supporting optimal kidney function.

Providing Education and Support: Renal dietitians are experts in the field of kidney health and nutrition. They possess in-depth knowledge of the latest research, dietary guidelines, and practical strategies for managing kidney disease through diet. They can educate you about the role of various nutrients, explain how certain foods may impact your kidney function, and provide guidance on portion control, meal planning, and food choices. Additionally, a renal dietitian can address any concerns or questions you may have, offering ongoing support and encouragement as you navigate your kidney-friendly diet. They can help you overcome challenges, adapt to changes in your condition, and make adjustments to your diet as needed.

Monitoring and Evaluating Progress: Working with a renal dietitian allows for regular monitoring and evaluation of your progress. As your lab results and health status evolve, your dietitian can reassess your nutritional needs and make necessary adjustments to your dietary plan. They can help you understand the impact of your diet on your lab results and overall health, empowering you to make informed decisions and take an active role in your kidney care. By maintaining an open line of communication with your dietitian and sharing your challenges and successes, you can continue to refine and optimize your kidney-friendly diet over time.

SETTING NUTRITION TARGETS WITH A RENAL DIETITIAN

By working closely with a renal dietitian, you will receive personalized nutrition targets that take into account your unique needs, medical history, lab results, and dietary preferences. These targets provide clear guidelines for the minimum and maximum amounts of each nutrient you should aim for in your daily intake. They serve as a roadmap to help you maintain a balanced and kidney-friendly diet.

To effectively track your adherence to these nutrition targets, the use of a food tracking app like Cronometer (Go.DadviceTV.com/app) is highly recommended. These apps allow you to log your meals, snacks, and beverages, and provide detailed information on the nutritional composition of the foods you consume. By recording your food intake and comparing it to your nutrition targets, you gain valuable insights into your dietary habits and can make adjustments as needed.

The beauty of setting nutrition targets and using a food tracking app is that they provide **flexibility and freedom** in your food choices. Within the framework of your targets, you have the freedom to select and enjoy a variety of foods. As long as you stay within your daily limits for calories, sodium, fiber, protein, potassium, iron, and other nutrients, you can tailor your meals according to your taste preferences and dietary needs.

Portion control and mindful eating are essential components of staying within your nutrition targets. These practices involve being mindful of your portion sizes and paying attention to your body's hunger and fullness cues. By practicing portion control, you can ensure that you consume appropriate amounts of food to meet your nutritional targets without overindulging or depriving yourself. Mindful eating encourages you to savor each bite, eat slowly, and fully engage with your food, promoting a healthier relationship with eating.

The combination of setting nutrition targets, using a food tracking app, practicing portion control, and adopting mindful eating habits forms a powerful strategy for managing your kidney-friendly diet. These practices provide structure, guidance, and accountability, while still allowing for flexibility and enjoyment of food. By adhering to your nutrition targets and incorporating portion control and mindful eating into your daily routine, you can cultivate a sustainable and health-promoting relationship with food.

Here is a form I use with my renal dietitian to set my daily nutritional targets:

	Daily Minimum		Daily Maximum	
Calories	_____________		_____________	
Calcium	_____________	mg	_____________	mg
Carbohydrates	_____________	grams	_____________	grams
Fiber	_____________	grams	_____________	grams
Iron	_____________	mg	_____________	mg
Protein	_____________	grams	_____________	grams
Phosphorus	_____________	mg	_____________	mg
Potassium	_____________	mg	_____________	mg
Sodium	_____________	mg	_____________	mg
Water	_____________	ounces	_____________	ounces
Avoid:	____			
Limit:	____			

MONITORING LAB RESULTS AND ADJUSTING

Monitoring lab results and adjusting your diet accordingly is a crucial aspect of the Dadvice TV Kidney Diet Strategy. By tracking your food intake using an app like Cronometer (Go.DadviceTV.com/app) and regularly reviewing your lab results, you gain valuable insights into the impact of your diet on your body's nutrient levels and overall kidney health.

Cronometer allows you to meticulously log your meals, snacks, and beverages, providing a comprehensive breakdown of the nutritional content of the foods you consume. This data becomes a valuable resource when you receive your next set of lab results, as it allows you to easily identify any values that fall outside the standard range.

For example, if your lab results indicate that your potassium levels are elevated, it is possible to review your food tracking app's report to see if you have exceeded your daily potassium targets. This information enables your dietitian to make informed decisions about adjusting your daily potassium targets to bring them back within a healthy range.

Regularly monitoring your lab results and comparing them to your nutrition targets helps you and your dietitian identify any areas that may require modification or additional attention. By pinpointing specific nutrients that may be problematic, such as potassium, sodium, or phosphorus, you can work collaboratively with your dietitian to make targeted adjustments to your diet.

If a particular nutrient is consistently outside the desired range, your dietitian may recommend specific dietary modifications to help you better manage your levels. These adjustments may involve reducing or increasing the consumption of certain foods or ingredients, implementing cooking techniques to leach out or reduce the content of specific nutrients, or making substitutions with lower nutrient alternatives.

Regular communication with your dietitian is essential in this process. By sharing your lab results and discussing your food tracking app's report, you create a collaborative environment where adjustments can be made based on your individual needs and circumstances. Your dietitian may provide further guidance on portion sizes, ingredient choices, meal planning, and cooking methods to help you maintain optimal nutrient levels and support your kidney health.

The synergy between monitoring lab results and utilizing a food tracking app like Cronometer allows you to make data-driven decisions about your diet. This approach empowers you to take an active role in managing your kidney health and provides you with a clear understanding of the impact of your dietary choices on your lab values.

By incorporating this monitoring and adjusting process into your kidney diet strategy, you can optimize your nutritional intake, maintain appropriate nutrient levels, and proactively manage your kidney health. This approach promotes a sense of empowerment, as you become an active participant in your care and gain a deeper understanding of how your diet impacts your overall well-being.

Remember, regular communication with your dietitian is vital in this process. Together, you can make informed decisions, fine-tune your dietary approach, and navigate the complexities of managing your kidney health with confidence and expertise.

Since my diagnosis of kidney failure, I have wholeheartedly embraced the Dadvice TV Kidney Diet Strategy and incorporated healthy lifestyle changes into my daily routine (as discussed in my book *Conquering Kidney Disease – A Survivor's Guide to Thriving with CKD*). For nearly five years, this strategy has served as the cornerstone of my journey to improved health, enhanced kidney function, and the elimination of all my kidney disease symptoms. By diligently adhering to the personalized nutrition targets set by my renal dietitian, tracking my food intake with Cronometer, and monitoring and adjusting based on my lab results, I have experienced firsthand the transformative power of a proactive approach to kidney health. The success I have achieved is a testament to the effectiveness of this strategy, and it is my sincere hope that by sharing my experiences and providing educational resources, others with kidney disease can also embark on a path of empowerment and thrive in their own health journey.

SODIUM: MASTERING SALT AND SODIUM INTAKE

In this chapter, we will explore the crucial role of sodium in kidney health and delve into effective strategies for reducing sodium intake in your diet. We will also discuss sodium alternatives and flavor enhancers that can be used to create delicious, low-sodium meals. Additionally, we will touch upon the different types of salt and their minor differences in sodium content, emphasizing that the majority of sodium in our diets comes from processed foods. Let's begin by understanding sodium's impact on kidney health.

UNDERSTANDING SODIUM'S IMPACT ON KIDNEY HEALTH

Sodium, a crucial mineral in our diets, plays a significant role in fluid balance and nerve and muscle function. However, excessive sodium intake can have detrimental effects on kidney health, particularly when it comes to managing high blood pressure, a common complication of kidney disease.

High blood pressure, or hypertension, places increased stress on the blood vessels and organs, including the kidneys. Over time, this heightened pressure can damage the delicate blood vessels within the kidneys and impair their ability to effectively filter waste products and regulate fluid balance. As a result, kidney function may decline, further exacerbating the progression of kidney disease.

Managing sodium intake is a vital component of managing high blood pressure and supporting kidney health at all stages of kidney disease. By reducing sodium consumption, individuals can help lower their blood pressure levels, alleviating the strain on the kidneys and potentially slowing the decline in kidney function.

While managing sodium intake is crucial at all stages of kidney disease, it becomes even more critical as kidney function declines. As the kidneys lose their filtering capacity, they struggle to excrete excess sodium, leading to fluid retention and increased blood pressure. This creates a vicious cycle where the impaired kidneys are further burdened by the effects of high blood pressure. Therefore, starting early and managing sodium intake from the onset of kidney disease can help slow the decline in kidney function and delay the need for interventions such as dialysis or transplantation.

However, managing sodium intake becomes more challenging as kidney function declines. The kidneys play a crucial role in regulating sodium balance, and as their function decreases, the ability to excrete sodium effectively becomes compromised. This means that individuals with advanced kidney disease need to be even more vigilant about their sodium intake to prevent fluid overload and further strain on the kidneys.

By adopting a proactive approach to managing sodium intake early on in the course of kidney disease, individuals can reduce the risk of high blood pressure, slow the decline in kidney function, and potentially improve their long-term kidney health outcomes. It is a small yet powerful step that can have a profound impact on overall kidney health and quality of life.

TIPS FOR REDUCING SODIUM IN YOUR DIET

Reducing sodium intake is an important aspect of a kidney-friendly diet. High sodium levels can contribute to fluid retention and increased blood pressure, which can put additional strain on the kidneys. Here are detailed tips and strategies for reducing sodium in your diet effectively.

Read Food Labels: Carefully reading food labels can help you identify hidden sources of sodium in packaged foods. Pay attention to the "Sodium" or "Na" value per serving and choose products with lower sodium content. Opt for products labeled as "low sodium" or "no added salt" whenever possible.

Limit Processed and Packaged Foods: Processed and packaged foods, including canned soups, frozen meals, deli meats, snacks, and condiments, tend to be high in sodium. Reduce your consumption of these foods and opt for fresh, whole foods instead. Cooking meals from scratch using fresh ingredients allows you to have better control over the amount of sodium added to your dishes.

Use Fresh Herbs and Spices: Enhance the flavor of your meals with fresh herbs and spices instead of relying on salt. Experiment with a variety of herbs like basil, oregano, thyme, and spices such as turmeric, cumin, paprika, or garlic powder. These can add depth and complexity to your dishes without the need for excessive sodium.

Choose Low-Sodium Ingredients: When shopping for ingredients, select low-sodium options. Look for low-sodium broths, sauces, and condiments, or consider making your own low-sodium versions at home. Be cautious of condiments like soy sauce, ketchup, and salad dressings, as they can be high in sodium. Look for low-sodium alternatives or make homemade versions with reduced sodium.

Cook from Scratch: Preparing meals at home gives you full control over the ingredients and allows you to reduce sodium content. Choose fresh, whole ingredients and cook using methods that enhance flavors, such as roasting, grilling, or sautéing with minimal added salt. Experiment with herbs, spices, and flavor-enhancing ingredients like citrus juice, vinegar, or low-sodium broths to add depth to your dishes.

Rinse Canned Foods: If using canned foods like beans or vegetables, rinsing them under running water can help reduce sodium content. Drain and rinse canned beans or vegetables before incorporating them into your recipes. This simple step can significantly decrease the sodium content by up to 40%.

Be Mindful of Hidden Sodium: Sodium can hide in unexpected places. Be cautious of foods labeled as "low fat" or "healthy," as they may compensate for reduced fat content by adding more sodium. Also, be mindful of sauces, gravies, and marinades, as they can be high in sodium. Consider making your own using low-sodium ingredients or using them sparingly. Plant-based meat substitutes are often loaded with sodium and can easily approach half of a day's sodium in a single serving.

Limit the Use of Salt in Cooking: Gradually reduce your reliance on salt while cooking. Use salt-free seasoning blends, herbs, and spices to add flavor instead. Over time, your taste buds will adjust, and you will become more sensitive to the natural flavors of foods.

Dine Out with Care: When eating out, request that your meal be prepared with minimal added salt or ask for dressings, sauces, and condiments to be served on the side. Choose steamed, grilled, or baked dishes over fried or heavily seasoned options. Many restaurants are accommodating to dietary requests, so don't hesitate to inquire about low-sodium alternatives.

Be Mindful of Sodium Substitutes: While sodium substitutes like potassium chloride-based salts can be an option for reducing sodium intake, they may not be suitable for individuals with certain health conditions, such as kidney disease or certain medications. It is important to consult with your healthcare team before incorporating sodium substitutes into your diet.

SODIUM ALTERNATIVES AND FLAVOR ENHANCERS FOR DELICIOUS, LOW-SODIUM MEALS

Reducing sodium intake doesn't mean sacrificing flavor. There are several sodium alternatives and flavor enhancers available that can add depth and richness to your meals without relying on excessive salt.

Herbs and Spices: Herbs and spices are a fantastic way to add robust flavors to your dishes. Experiment with a wide variety of options such as basil, oregano, thyme, rosemary, cumin, turmeric, paprika, ginger, and cinnamon. These aromatic ingredients can elevate the taste profile of your meals, making them flavorful and satisfying.

Citrus Juices and Zests: Freshly squeezed lemon, lime, or orange juice can provide a tangy and refreshing flavor to your dishes. Add citrus juice to dressings, marinades, sauces, and seafood dishes for a burst of brightness. You can also grate the zest of citrus fruits to add a zingy essence to your cooking.

Vinegars: Various types of vinegar, such as balsamic, apple cider, rice, or red wine vinegar, can bring a tangy and acidic taste to your recipes. Use them in salad dressings, marinades, pickles, and sauces to enhance the overall flavor profile of your dishes.

Aromatics: Aromatics like onions, garlic, shallots, and leeks can provide depth and complexity to your cooking. Sautéing or caramelizing these ingredients can bring out their natural sweetness and savory qualities. They serve as a flavor base for many recipes, adding richness without relying heavily on salt.

Low-Sodium Broths and Stocks: Opt for low-sodium or no-salt-added broths and stocks to infuse depth into soups, stews, and sauces. These flavorful liquids can add complexity to your dishes without overwhelming them with sodium. You can also make your own broths using fresh ingredients and herbs.

Salt-Free Seasoning Blends: Explore salt-free seasoning blends available in stores or create your own by combining various herbs, spices, and other flavorings. These blends often include a combination of ingredients like garlic powder, onion powder, paprika, dried herbs, and other aromatic spices. They can be used as a convenient and flavorful alternative to salt.

Umami-Enhancing Ingredients: Umami is known as the fifth taste, characterized as a savory, meaty, or earthy flavor. Incorporate umami-rich ingredients like mushrooms, tomatoes, miso paste, nutritional yeast, soy sauce alternatives (such as low-sodium tamari or coconut aminos), or fermented foods like kimchi or sauerkraut to add depth and complexity to your dishes.

Roasting and Grilling: Cooking techniques like roasting and grilling can intensify the flavors of foods naturally. The caramelization process adds depth and richness to vegetables, proteins, and even fruits. Roasted or grilled ingredients can be a flavorful centerpiece or complement to your meals.

Homemade Sauces and Dressings: Prepare your own sauces, dressings, and condiments using low-sodium ingredients. Experiment with combinations of vinegars, citrus juices, herbs, spices, mustard, yogurt, or olive oil to create flavorful accompaniments that enhance the taste of your dishes.

Taste and Adjust: As you reduce your sodium intake, your taste buds will become more sensitive to subtle flavors. Embrace the journey of discovering new tastes and adjust seasonings accordingly. Taste your dishes as you cook and make necessary adjustments with herbs, spices, acids, or other flavor-enhancing ingredients to achieve the desired balance of flavors.

DELICIOUS SEASONING COMBOS

- Asparagus: Garlic, Lemon Juice, Onion, Vinegar
- Beef: Basil, Bay Leaf, Chilis, Coriander, Garlic, Green Pepper, Marjoram, Mushrooms, Mustard, Nutmeg, Onion, Oregano, Parsley, Pepper, Safe, Tarragon, Thyme
- Bread: Anise, Basil, Caraway, Cardamom, Cinnamon, Cloves, Cumin, Dill, Lemon Peel, Poppy Seeds, Saffron, Sesame Seeds
- Broccoli: Lemon Juice, Garlic
- Cheese: Caraway, Celery Seed, Chervil, Chives, Curry,

Dill, Garlic, Horseradish, Lemon Peel, Mustard, Nutmeg, Parsley, Pepper, Sage

- Chicken: Allspice, Basil, Bay Leaf, Cinnamon, Curry, Dill, Garlic, Ginger, Lime, Lemon, Marjoram, Mushrooms, Oregano, Paprika, Parsley, Poultry Seasoning, Saffron, Sage, Tarragon, Thyme
- Cucumbers: Chives, Dill, Garlic, Onion, Vinegar
- Eggs: Basil, Chervil, Chives, Curry, Dill, Fennel, Ginger, Paprika, Parsley, Pepper, Sage, Tarragon
- Fish: Basil, Bay Leaf, Chives, Curry, Dill, Fennel, Garlic, Ginger, Lemon, Mustard, Paprika, Parsley, Tarragon
- Fruit: Allspice, Anise, Cardamom, Cinnamon, Cloves, Coriander, Ginger, Mint, Nutmeg
- Green Beans: Dill, Lemon Juice, Nutmeg, Marjoram
- Greens: Onion, Pepper, Vinegar
- Lamb: Basil, Bay Leaf, Cinnamon, Coriander, Cumin, Curry, Dill, Garlic, Mint, Parsley, Pineapple, Rosemary, Tarragon, Thyme
- Pasta: Basil, Caraway Seed, Garlic, Oregano, Poppy Seed
- Peas: Green Pepper, Mint, Parsley, Onion, Fresh Mushrooms
- Pork: Apple, Applesauce, Garlic, Onion, Sage
- Potatoes: Green Pepper, Mace, Onion, Paprika, Parsley
- Rice: Chives, Green Pepper, Saffron, Onion
- Salad Dressings: Basil, Chives, Dill, Fennel, Garlic, Horseradish, Mustard, Oregano, Paprika, Parsley, Saffron, Tarragon
- Salads: Basil, Chives, Dill, Garlic, Lemon, Mint, Oregano, Parsley, Tarragon
- Salt Substitutes: Allspice, Basil, Bay Leaf,

Caraway, Cardamom, Curry, Dash, Dill, Ginger, Marjoram, Rosemary, Thyme, Safe, Tarragon

- Soups (Homemade): Basil, Bay Leaf, Chervil, Chilis, Chives, Cumin, Dill, Fennel, Garlic, Parsley, Pepper, Rosemary, Sage, Thyme
- Squash: Cinnamon, Nutmeg, Mace, Ginger
- Sweets: Allspice, Anise, Cardamom, Cinnamon, Cloves, Fennel, Lemon Peel, Ginger, Mace, Nutmeg, Mint
- Tomatoes: Basil, Marjoram, Onion, Oregano,
- Veal: Apricot, Cinnamon, Cloves, Ginger

It's worth mentioning that the differences between various types of salt, such as sea salt, kosher salt, and table salt, are relatively minor in terms of sodium content. The majority of sodium in our diets actually comes from processed foods rather than table salt used during cooking or at the table. Therefore, focusing on reducing the consumption of processed and packaged foods is crucial in lowering overall sodium intake.

Personally, I prefer using Pink Himalayan Sea Salt in a grinder. This allows me to have better control over the amount of salt I add to my meals, as the grinding process makes me more aware of the quantity. However, it's important to note that the choice of salt is a personal preference, and what matters most is the overall reduction in sodium intake from all sources.

By being mindful of the sodium content in the foods we consume and incorporating these sodium-reducing strategies into our daily routines, we can make significant strides in managing our sodium intake and supporting kidney health.

Remember, while sodium plays a role in flavor enhancement,

there are numerous alternatives and creative ways to make delicious, low-sodium meals. By exploring these options and embracing the natural flavors of fresh ingredients, you can create satisfying dishes that nourish your body and support your kidney-healthy lifestyle.

POTASSIUM: BALANCING ELECTROLYTES

In this chapter, we will explore the important role of potassium in kidney health and delve into strategies for managing potassium levels through food choices. We will discuss potassium-rich foods, provide tips for moderating potassium intake, and clarify when potassium restriction may be necessary. It is important to note that while potassium is generally beneficial and protective for the heart and kidneys, restrictions may be needed based on individual circumstances, as determined by your healthcare team or dietitian. Additionally, certain medications can impact potassium levels, requiring careful monitoring. Let's begin by understanding the role of potassium in kidney health.

THE ROLE OF POTASSIUM IN KIDNEY HEALTH

Potassium is an essential mineral that plays a vital role in maintaining proper cell function, nerve transmission, and muscle contractions, including the heart muscle. In the context of kidney health, potassium is particularly important because the kidneys regulate potassium levels in the body. Healthy kidneys help to maintain a delicate balance of potassium by excreting excess amounts through urine.

Adequate potassium intake is generally beneficial and protective for the heart and kidneys. Potassium helps counteract the effects of sodium, promoting healthy blood pressure levels and reducing the risk of hypertension, a common complication of kidney disease. It also supports proper muscle function, including the heart muscle, which is critical for maintaining cardiovascular health.

SYMPTOMS OF TOO MUCH AND TOO LITTLE POTASSIUM

Maintaining the right balance of potassium in your body is crucial for optimal health. Both excessively high and low levels of potassium can have adverse effects on various bodily functions. Here are some symptoms to be aware of:

Symptoms of Hyperkalemia (Too Much Potassium):

When potassium levels rise above the normal range, a condition known as hyperkalemia, it can have detrimental effects on the body. Symptoms of hyperkalemia may include:

- Irregular heartbeat or palpitations
- Muscle weakness or cramps
- Nausea and vomiting
- Fatigue or weakness
- Tingling or numbness
- Difficulty breathing
- Digestive disturbances

If you experience any of these symptoms, it is essential to seek medical attention promptly, as hyperkalemia can be life-threatening.

Symptoms of Hypokalemia (Too Little Potassium):

Conversely, low levels of potassium, known as hypokalemia, can also have adverse effects on your health. Symptoms of hypokalemia may include:

- Muscle weakness or cramps
- Fatigue or weakness
- Irregular heartbeat or palpitations
- Constipation
- Tingling or numbness
- Increased urination
- Feeling faint or lightheaded

If you suspect you have low potassium levels and experience these symptoms, it is important to consult with your healthcare team for proper evaluation and management.

MANAGING POTASSIUM LEVELS THROUGH FOOD CHOICES

Managing potassium levels involves making mindful food choices. By selecting appropriate foods and portion sizes, individuals can help regulate their potassium intake. Here are some strategies for managing potassium through dietary choices:

Identify Potassium-Rich Foods: Understanding which foods are high in potassium is essential for managing intake. Examples of potassium-rich foods include bananas, oranges, tomatoes, potatoes, avocados, spinach, and certain legumes. By being aware of these sources, you can make informed decisions about portion sizes and frequency of consumption.

Portion Control: Controlling portion sizes is crucial to manage potassium intake effectively. For foods high in potassium, such as those mentioned above, moderate portions are generally recommended. This allows for enjoyment of these nutritious foods while preventing excessive potassium intake.

Cooking Techniques: Some cooking techniques can help reduce the potassium content in certain foods. Leaching or soaking vegetables and fruits in water before cooking can help decrease their potassium levels. Boiling and discarding the cooking water can also remove some of the potassium from foods.

Diversify Your Diet: A varied diet that includes a range of food groups can help distribute potassium intake more evenly. Incorporating a wide variety of fruits, vegetables, whole grains, lean proteins, and healthy fats can provide a balanced nutritional profile while managing potassium levels.

POTASSIUM-RICH FOODS AND TIPS FOR MODERATING INTAKE

While potassium is generally beneficial, there are instances where potassium intake needs to be moderated. This typically occurs when the kidneys are no longer able to effectively regulate potassium levels. Your healthcare team or registered dietitian will inform you if a potassium restriction is necessary and provide you with specific daily minimum and maximum targets tailored to your individual needs.

When a potassium restriction is required, it is essential to be mindful of foods high in potassium and limit their consumption. Along with the previously mentioned potassium-rich foods, other examples include dried fruits, melons, kiwis, certain citrus fruits, and some types of beans. Preparing meals with lower potassium alternatives and incorporating variety in your diet can help ensure adequate nutrition while managing potassium intake.

It is important to note that medications can also impact potassium levels. Some medications, such as certain diuretics and potassium-sparing medications, can affect potassium balance in the body. Close monitoring of potassium levels and regular communication with your healthcare team are crucial if you are taking such medications.

WHEN TO RESTRICT POTASSIUM

Potassium restriction becomes necessary when lab results indicate that your kidneys are no longer effectively managing potassium levels. This typically occurs in advanced stages of kidney disease or when specific medical conditions require tighter control of potassium intake. Your healthcare team or registered dietitian will closely monitor your lab results and provide guidance on when to restrict potassium.

When potassium restriction is advised, your healthcare team will provide you with a daily minimum and maximum target for potassium intake. It is important to adhere to these recommendations to prevent potassium imbalances that can lead to complications.

It is worth noting that potassium restriction does not mean complete elimination of potassium-rich foods from your diet. Instead, it involves moderation and careful portion control. Working with a registered dietitian who specializes in kidney health will help you create a personalized meal plan that meets your nutritional needs while managing potassium intake effectively.

By monitoring your potassium levels, following dietary recommendations, and working closely with your healthcare team, you can maintain a healthy balance of potassium and support kidney health.

Remember, managing potassium levels is an important aspect of your overall kidney health. The majority of individuals with kidney disease can benefit from potassium-rich foods as part of a balanced diet. However, restrictions may be necessary for some individuals based on their specific medical conditions and stage of kidney disease. Always consult with your healthcare team or registered dietitian for personalized recommendations and guidance.

PHOSPHORUS: CONTROLLING PHOSPHORUS LEVELS

In this chapter, we will explore the importance of managing phosphorus levels in kidney disease and delve into strategies for controlling phosphorus intake. We will discuss low-phosphorus food choices, how to read labels and identify phosphorus additives, the difference between natural phosphorus and phosphorus additives in terms of absorption, and the role of phosphorus binders in controlling phosphorus absorption. Understanding these aspects will empower you to take an active role in managing your phosphorus levels effectively. Let's begin by understanding the significance of phosphorus management in kidney disease.

IMPORTANCE OF PHOSPHORUS MANAGEMENT IN KIDNEY DISEASE

Phosphorus is an essential mineral that plays a vital role in various bodily functions, including bone health, energy production, and cell function. However, in kidney disease, the kidneys are less able to regulate phosphorus levels, leading to an accumulation of phosphorus in the blood.

Elevated blood phosphorus levels, known as hyperphosphatemia, can contribute to complications such as bone and cardiovascular problems. Excessive phosphorus in the blood can lead to the release of calcium from the bones, weakening them over time. Additionally, high phosphorus levels can trigger the release of hormones that negatively affect blood vessels, potentially increasing the risk of cardiovascular disease.

Managing phosphorus levels is crucial in preventing these complications and supporting overall kidney health. By controlling phosphorus intake, individuals with kidney disease can help maintain a balance and minimize the risks associated with hyperphosphatemia.

LOW-PHOSPHORUS FOOD CHOICES AND STRATEGIES

Controlling phosphorus intake involves making smart food choices and adopting strategies to limit phosphorus-rich foods. Here are some tips for managing phosphorus levels:

Choose Low-Phosphorus Foods: Focus on incorporating foods that are naturally low in phosphorus into your diet. Examples include fresh fruits and vegetables, lean proteins such as chicken, fish, and egg whites, whole grains, and healthy fats like olive oil and avocado.

Limit Phosphorus-Rich Foods: Certain foods are naturally high in phosphorus and should be limited or avoided. These include dairy products, such as milk, cheese, and yogurt, processed meats, whole grains, dried beans, and nuts. Working with your healthcare team or registered dietitian can help you identify specific foods to limit based on your individual needs.

Cooking Techniques: Some cooking techniques, such as soaking or leaching certain foods, can help reduce their phosphorus content. For example, soaking beans before cooking or leaching vegetables in water can help remove some of the phosphorus.

Portion Control: Controlling portion sizes is essential for managing phosphorus intake. Even foods that are relatively low in phosphorus can contribute to overall intake if consumed in large amounts. Moderation is key to maintaining a healthy balance.

Common Low Phosphorus Foods:

Category	Food	Serving Size	Phosphorus Content (mg)
Meat or Poultry	Beef, pot roast	3 ounces	155
	Beef, sirloin steak	3 ounces	195
	Chicken breast	3 ounces	180
	Chicken thigh, skinless	3 ounces	150
	Hamburger patty, 90% lean	3 ounces	170
	Lamb chops	3 ounces	160
	Lean ground beef	3 ounces	180
	Pork chop	3 ounces	200

Category	Food	Serving	Phosphorus
	Pork roast	3 ounces	190
	Pork tenderloin	3 ounces	180
	Turkey breast	3 ounces	185
	Turkey thigh meat, skinless	3 ounces	170
	Veal chop	3 ounces	200
Seafood	Cod	3 ounces	75
	King crab	3 ounces	192
	Lobster	3 ounces	160
	Mahi Mahi	3 ounces	155
	Oysters, Eastern	3 ounces	120
	Rockfish	3 ounces	195
	Salmon	3 ounces	230
	Sea bass	3 ounces	210
	Shrimp	3 ounces	130
	Snow crab	3 ounces	120
	Tilapia	3 ounces	150
	Tuna (canned in water)	3 ounces	175
	Yellowfin tuna	3 ounces	210

		Size	Content (mg)
Bread	Bagel: blueberry	1 medium	70
	Bagel: cinnamon raisin	1 medium	70
	Bagel: onion	1 medium	70
	Bagel: plain	1 medium	70
	Brown rice	1/2 cup	40
	Corn tortilla, 6-inch	1 tortilla	75
	English muffin	1 muffin	76
	Flatbread	1 piece	48
	Flour tortillas, no baking powder	1 tortilla	37
	French or Italian bread or rolls	1 slice	29

	Light wheat bread	1 slice	38
	Oatmeal	1/2 cup	80
	Pita bread, white	1 pita	58
	Quinoa	1/2 cup	100
	Sourdough bread	1 slice	30
	White bread	1 slice	25
	Whole wheat bread	1 slice	50
	Whole wheat pasta	1/2 cup	70
Pasta or Rice	Couscous	1/2 cup	20
	Egg noodles	1/2 cup	60
	Macaroni	1/2 cup	40
	Pearled barley	1/2 cup	43
	Plain white rice, short, medium, or long	1/2 cup	35
	Rice noodles	1/2	28

		cup	
	Spaghetti	1/2 cup	42
Dairy or Dairy Substitutes	Almond milk	1 cup	150
	Almond milk, Almond Breeze®, original	1/2 cup	50
	Cottage cheese	1/2 cup	80
	Egg whites, pasteurized	1/2 cup	15
	Greek yogurt	1 cup	150
	Nondairy creamer without phosphate additives	1/2 cup	53
	Nondairy whipped topping	2 tbsp	10
	Sherbet	1/2 cup	38
	Sour cream	2 tbsp	40
	Soy milk	1 cup	150
	Unenriched rice milk without calcium-phosphate	1/2 cup	29

Category	Food	Serving Size	Phosphorus Content (mg)
	Unsweetened yogurt	1 cup	200

Category	Food	Serving Size	Phosphorus Content (mg)
Snack Foods	Applesauce	1/2 cup	6
	Baby carrots	9 pieces	25
	Blueberries	1/2 cup	9
	Celery	1 stalk	10
	Cherries	1/2 cup	15
	Fig bar	2 bars	25
	Fruit candies: hard, chews or gummy	-	0
	Fruit cocktail	1/2 cup	17
	Low-sodium crackers	1 ounce	35
	Peach, 1 medium	1	10

		medium	
	Pineapple	1/2 cup	6
	Popcorn (air-popped)	3 cups	45
	Pretzels	1 ounce	60
	Radishes	1	9
	Rice cakes	1 cake	20
	Strawberries, fresh	1/2 cup	18
	Unsalted almonds	1 ounce	160
	Unsalted peanuts	1 ounce	130
	Unsalted popcorn	1 cup	8
	Unsalted pretzels	1 ounce	40
Fruits and Vegetables	Apples	1 medium	20
	Spinach	1/2	20

		cup	
	Bell peppers	1 medium	20
	Broccoli	1/2 cup	30
	Cauliflower	1/2 cup	15
Cheese	Blue cheese	1 ounce	110
	Cottage cheese	1/4 cup	92
	Cream cheese	1 ounce	40
	Cream cheese	2 tbsp	40
	Feta cheese	1 ounce	130
	Feta cheese	1 ounce	96
	Mozzarella cheese	1 ounce	200
	Neufchatel cheese	1 ounce	39

		e	
	Parmesan cheese, grated	2 tbsp	72
	Ricotta cheese	1 ounce	35
	Swiss cheese	1 ounce	110

HOW TO READ LABELS AND IDENTIFY PHOSPHORUS ADDITIVES

Reading food labels carefully can help identify phosphorus additives in processed and packaged foods. Look for terms such as phosphoric acid, sodium phosphate, calcium phosphate, and other similar additives. These additives can significantly contribute to your phosphorus intake, so it is important to be aware of their presence and limit consumption accordingly. One trick I like is looking for PHOS in the ingredients list. If it appears more than once in the first half of the ingredients, or more than twice in total, then I avoid the product.

Here are some common phosphorus additives:
- Aluminum **phos**phate
- Dicalcium **phos**phate
- Hexameta**phos**phate
- Monocalcium **phos**phate

- **Phos**phoric acid
- Poly**phos**phate
- Pyro**phos**phate
- Sodium poly**phos**phate
- Sodium tripoly**phos**phate
- Tetrasodium **phos**phate
- Tricalcium **phos**phate
- Trisodium **phos**phate

THE DIFFERENCE IN ABSORPTION OF NATURAL PHOSPHORUS VS. PHOSPHORUS ADDITIVES

It is worth noting that the body absorbs phosphorus from natural food sources differently compared to phosphorus additives found in processed foods. Natural phosphorus found in whole foods is typically absorbed at a lower rate by the body compared to phosphorus additives, which are readily absorbed. This difference underscores the importance of focusing on whole, unprocessed foods and minimizing the consumption of processed and packaged items. Here are the approximate absorption rates by category:

Organic phosphorus found in grains: The absorption percentage of organic phosphorus from grains can vary depending on factors such as the form of phosphorus and the presence of other compounds in the food. According to a study published in the Journal of Nutrition, the absorption of organic phosphorus from grains ranges from approximately 40% to 60% (Coudray et al., 2005). However, it's important to note that the bioavailability of phosphorus from plant-based sources can be lower due to the presence of phytic acid and other compounds that can bind phosphorus and reduce its absorption.

Organic phosphorus found in nuts & meat: The absorption of organic phosphorus from nuts and meat can vary depending on factors such as the specific type of nut or meat and individual differences. The bioavailability of phosphorus from animal-based sources, such as meat, poultry, and fish, is generally higher compared to plant-based sources. According to a study published in the Journal of Nutrition, the absorption of organic phosphorus from animal sources can range from approximately 50% to 70% (Hunt et al., 2009). Nuts, on the other hand, may have varying levels of bioavailability depending on the type of nut and the presence of compounds that can affect phosphorus absorption.

Organic phosphorus found in dairy: The absorption of organic phosphorus from dairy products is generally high due to the presence of phosphorus in a highly bioavailable form. According to a review published in the Journal of Renal Nutrition, the absorption of organic phosphorus from dairy products can range from approximately 70% to 90% (Dhaene et al., 2012). However, it's important to note that individuals with kidney disease may need to monitor their intake of dairy products due to their phosphorus content.

Inorganic phosphorus: Inorganic phosphorus additives, commonly found in processed and packaged foods, are generally well absorbed by the body. The bioavailability of inorganic phosphorus can be as high as 100%. These additives, such as phosphoric acid or sodium phosphate, are more easily absorbed by the body compared to organic phosphorus from whole foods. However, it's important to note that excessive intake of inorganic phosphorus can be detrimental to kidney health, especially in individuals with kidney disease.

Common phosphorus additives (look for PHOS in the ingredients):
· Aluminum **phos**phate
· Dicalcium **phos**phate

- Hexameta**phos**phate
- Monocalcium **phos**phate
- **Phos**phoric acid
- Poly**phos**phate
- Pyro**phos**phate
- Sodium poly**phos**phate
- Sodium tripoly**phos**phate
- Tetrasodium **phos**phate
- Tricalcium **phos**phate
- Trisodium **phos**phate

It's worth mentioning that the absorption percentages mentioned above are approximate ranges based on available scientific research. The actual absorption of phosphorus can vary among individuals and may be influenced by factors such as overall diet, individual health conditions, and the presence of other nutrients or compounds that can affect phosphorus absorption.

References:

Coudray, C., Feillet-Coudray, C., Tressol, J. C., Gueux, E., Thulk, J. C., & Mazur, A. (2005). Phytic acid and mineral bioavailability. The Journal of Nutrition, 135(9), 2369-2372.

Hunt, J. R., Johnson, L. K., Fariba Roughead, Z., & Lykken, G. I. (2009). How stable is the mineral content of the food supply? Journal of Food Composition and Analysis, 22(5), 382-388.

Dhaene, M., Leroy, B., Snauwaert, E., & Vervaet, B. A. (2012). Dietary phosphate intake in chronic kidney disease: Review of phosphorus additives. Journal of Renal Nutrition, 22(2), 195-199.

PHOSPHORUS BINDERS AND THEIR ROLE IN CONTROLLING PHOSPHORUS ABSORPTION

Phosphorus binders are medications that can help control phosphorus absorption in individuals with kidney disease. These binders work by binding to dietary phosphorus in the digestive tract, preventing its absorption into the bloodstream. By reducing the amount of phosphorus absorbed, phosphorus binders help maintain healthy phosphorus levels.

Phosphorus binders are typically taken with meals or snacks, as this is when phosphorus from food is ingested. They come in various forms, such as chewable tablets, capsules, or powders, and are available in different strengths. Your healthcare team or registered dietitian will determine the appropriate type, dosage, and timing of phosphorus binders based on your individual needs and phosphorus levels.

It's important to note that phosphorus binders should be taken as directed and not as a substitute for a low-phosphorus diet. They are intended to complement dietary strategies and provide additional support in controlling phosphorus absorption.

By working closely with your healthcare team, registered dietitian, and following their recommendations, you can effectively manage phosphorus levels and reduce the risks associated with elevated phosphorus in kidney disease. Regular monitoring of blood phosphorus levels and close communication with your healthcare team will help ensure that your phosphorus management plan is personalized and optimized for your specific needs.

In the next chapter, we will explore the role of protein in kidney health and discuss guidelines for managing protein intake to support your kidney function while meeting your nutritional needs. Understanding the nuances of protein intake will empower you to make informed choices that optimize your kidney health journey.

PROTEIN: MODERATION FOR KIDNEY HEALTH

In this chapter, we will delve into the role of protein in kidney disease and explore strategies for moderating protein intake while ensuring adequate nutrition. We will discuss high-quality protein sources, portion control recommendations, and the impact of animal protein versus plant-based protein on kidney health. Understanding these aspects will empower you to make informed choices that optimize your kidney health. Let's begin by understanding the role of protein in kidney disease.

UNDERSTANDING PROTEIN'S ROLE IN KIDNEY DISEASE

Protein is an essential macronutrient that plays a crucial role in various bodily functions, including tissue repair, immune function, and hormone production. However, in the context of kidney disease, protein needs to be moderated to reduce the burden on the kidneys.

When protein is digested and metabolized, it produces waste products, including urea and other nitrogenous compounds. The kidneys are responsible for filtering and excreting these waste products from the bloodstream. In individuals with compromised kidney function, the kidneys may have difficulty processing and eliminating excessive protein waste, potentially leading to further kidney damage.

Signs of Too Much Protein in Your Diet

Digestive Issues: Consuming excessive protein can put a strain on your digestive system, leading to symptoms such as bloating, gas, constipation, or diarrhea.

Dehydration: High-protein diets can increase fluid needs, and if adequate hydration is not maintained, it can lead to dehydration. Signs of dehydration include dark urine, dry mouth, thirst, and fatigue.

Kidney Stress: Excessive protein intake can put additional stress on the kidneys, particularly in individuals with compromised kidney function. Signs of kidney stress may include changes in urine output, frequent urination, or discomfort in the kidney area.

Bad Breath: When protein is broken down, it produces ammonia as a waste product. Consuming excessive protein can result in an ammonia-like odor on the breath, commonly referred to as "ketosis breath."

Signs of Too Little Protein in Your Diet

Muscle Weakness: Protein is essential for building and maintaining muscle tissue. Inadequate protein intake may lead to muscle weakness, loss of muscle mass, and decreased strength.

Fatigue and Low Energy Levels: Protein provides energy and supports various bodily functions. Insufficient protein intake can result in low energy levels, persistent fatigue, and difficulty concentrating.

Poor Wound Healing: Protein plays a crucial role in tissue repair and wound healing. If your diet lacks adequate protein, you may experience slower healing of wounds, injuries, or surgical incisions.

Hair, Skin, and Nail Issues: Protein is essential for the health and maintenance of hair, skin, and nails. Inadequate protein intake can result in brittle hair, dry skin, and weak or brittle nails.

Impaired Immune Function: Protein is necessary for the production of antibodies and enzymes involved in immune function. Insufficient protein intake may weaken the immune system, making you more susceptible to infections or illnesses.

It's important to note that these signs may not be exclusive to protein intake alone and can be influenced by other factors. If you suspect you are experiencing issues related to protein intake, it is advisable to consult with your healthcare team or registered dietitian for a comprehensive assessment and personalized guidance based on your individual needs.

STRATEGIES FOR MODERATING PROTEIN INTAKE WHILE MEETING NUTRITIONAL NEEDS

Moderating protein intake is important to reduce the workload on the kidneys while still meeting your nutritional needs. Here are some strategies for achieving this balance:

Individualized Protein Recommendations: Work closely with your healthcare team or registered dietitian to determine your personalized protein requirements based on your kidney function, nutritional status, and other individual factors. Protein needs can vary depending on the stage of kidney disease, level of kidney function, and presence of other health conditions.

Focus on High-Quality Protein Sources: Choose high-quality protein sources that provide essential amino acids while minimizing the intake of excess fat, cholesterol, and phosphorus. Examples of high-quality protein sources include lean meats, poultry, fish, eggs, low-fat dairy products, and plant-based protein sources such as legumes, tofu, tempeh, and quinoa.

Portion Control: Pay attention to portion sizes to manage protein intake effectively. Moderation is key, and balancing the quantity of protein with other macronutrients is crucial. Your healthcare team or registered dietitian can provide guidance on appropriate portion sizes based on your individual needs.

Distribution of Protein Intake: Spreading protein intake evenly throughout the day, rather than consuming large amounts in a single meal, can be beneficial. This distribution helps optimize protein utilization and minimizes the workload on the kidneys.

HIGH-QUALITY PROTEIN SOURCES AND PORTION CONTROL RECOMMENDATIONS

When selecting protein sources, it is important to focus on high-quality options that provide essential nutrients while being mindful of portion sizes. Here are some recommendations:

Lean Meats and Poultry: Choose lean cuts of meat and poultry, removing visible fat before cooking. Recommended portion sizes typically range from 3 to 4 ounces (85 to 113 grams) per meal.

Fish: Opt for fatty fish rich in omega-3 fatty acids, such as salmon, mackerel, and sardines. Portion sizes can vary, but a general guideline is around 3 to 4 ounces (85 to 113 grams) per meal.

Eggs: Include eggs as a protein source, focusing on the egg whites. One large egg contains around 6 grams of protein. Consult with your healthcare team or registered dietitian for personalized recommendations.

Low-Fat Dairy Products: Choose low-fat or fat-free dairy products, such as skim milk, low-fat yogurt, and reduced-fat cheese. Portion sizes for dairy products may vary, so it's important to refer to nutrition labels and follow recommendations from your healthcare team or registered dietitian.

Plant-Based Protein Sources: Include plant-based protein sources such as legumes (beans, lentils, chickpeas), tofu, tempeh, and quinoa. These options provide protein while offering additional nutritional benefits such as fiber, vitamins, and minerals. Portion sizes for plant-based proteins may vary, so it's important to consider the specific food and follow recommendations from your healthcare team or registered dietitian.

THE IMPACT OF ANIMAL PROTEIN VS. PLANT-BASED PROTEIN ON KIDNEY HEALTH

When considering the impact of animal protein and plant-based protein on kidney health, it's important to note some key differences. Animal protein sources, such as meat, poultry, and dairy products, tend to be higher in phosphorus and can potentially put more stress on the kidneys.

Animal protein digestion produces more acid, leading to increased acid load in the body. To maintain a balanced pH, the body may utilize a process called hyperfiltration, which involves increased blood flow to the kidneys. Over time, this increased workload on the kidneys can be taxing, potentially contributing to the progression of kidney disease and decline of kidney function.

On the other hand, plant-based protein sources generally have a lower phosphorus content and can help reduce the acid load on the body. Additionally, plant-based proteins are often accompanied by dietary fiber, which can have additional health benefits, including improved digestion and blood sugar control.

While plant-based protein sources offer potential advantages, it's important to note that individual needs may vary. Some individuals may tolerate animal protein sources well, while others may benefit from incorporating more plant-based proteins. Your healthcare team or registered dietitian can help you determine the most suitable protein sources based on your specific health needs and kidney function.

By balancing protein intake, choosing high-quality protein

sources, and being mindful of portion sizes, you can optimize your protein intake while supporting your kidney health. Remember, moderation is key, and individualized recommendations are essential in managing protein intake effectively.

In the next chapter, we will explore the role of fiber in kidney health and discuss its importance, sources, and strategies for incorporating fiber-rich foods into your kidney-healthy diet. Understanding the benefits of fiber will empower you to make dietary choices that support your overall well-being and kidney function.

FIBER: SUPPORTING DIGESTIVE HEALTH

In this chapter, we will explore the role of fiber in supporting digestive health for individuals with kidney disease. We will discuss the benefits of fiber, kidney-friendly high-fiber foods, the use of fiber supplements, and how to balance fiber intake with other dietary considerations. Understanding the importance of fiber and its impact on kidney health will empower you to make informed choices that support your overall well-being. Let's begin by understanding the benefits of fiber for kidney disease patients.

THE BENEFITS OF FIBER FOR KIDNEY DISEASE PATIENTS

Fiber offers several benefits for individuals with kidney disease, including:

Digestive Health: Fiber plays a crucial role in maintaining regular bowel movements, preventing constipation, and supporting overall digestive health. This is particularly important for individuals with kidney disease, as they may be more prone to constipation due to factors such as reduced physical activity, certain medications, or inadequate fluid intake.

Blood Sugar Control: High-fiber foods help slow down the absorption of glucose, promoting better blood sugar control. This can be beneficial for individuals with diabetes, a common condition associated with kidney disease.

Heart Health: A fiber-rich diet has been linked to a reduced risk of cardiovascular disease, which is a major concern for individuals with kidney disease. Fiber helps lower cholesterol levels, improve blood pressure, and promote overall heart health.

Weight Management: Fiber-rich foods tend to be more filling, which can help control appetite and support weight management. Maintaining a healthy weight is important for individuals with kidney disease, as excess weight can contribute to the progression of kidney disease and increase the risk of complications.

Signs of Too Little or Too Much Fiber in Your Diet:

Too Little Fiber: Signs of insufficient fiber intake may include constipation, irregular bowel movements, and difficulty passing stools. Inadequate fiber intake can also contribute to increased hunger, poor blood sugar control, and a higher risk of cardiovascular disease.

Too Much Fiber: Excessive fiber intake can cause bloating, gas, abdominal discomfort, and diarrhea. It is important to gradually increase fiber intake to allow the digestive system to adapt and ensure proper hydration to support healthy digestion.

KIDNEY-FRIENDLY HIGH-FIBER FOODS AND THEIR IMPORTANCE

Including kidney-friendly high-fiber foods in your diet can provide numerous health benefits. Here are some examples:

Whole Grains: Opt for whole grains such as brown rice, whole wheat bread, quinoa, and oats. These grains are rich in dietary fiber, vitamins, minerals, and antioxidants.

Fruits and Vegetables: Incorporate a variety of fruits and vegetables, such as berries, apples, oranges, broccoli, cauliflower, bell peppers, and leafy greens. These foods provide not only fiber but also essential nutrients vital for overall health.

Legumes: Include legumes like beans, lentils, and chickpeas in your meals. They are excellent sources of fiber, protein, and other important nutrients.

Nuts and Seeds: Enjoy moderate portions of nuts and seeds, such as almonds, walnuts, chia seeds, and flaxseeds. They provide fiber, healthy fats, and micronutrients.

Psyllium Husk: Psyllium husk is a soluble fiber supplement that can be added to foods or beverages to increase fiber intake. Consult with your healthcare team or registered dietitian before incorporating any fiber supplements into your routine.

FIBER SUPPLEMENTS FOR KIDNEY PATIENTS

Fiber supplements may be beneficial for individuals who struggle to meet their daily fiber needs through diet alone. However, it is important to consult with your healthcare team or registered dietitian before starting any fiber supplement. They can guide you on appropriate supplement choices, dosage, and potential interactions with your current medications or medical conditions.

Fiber supplements commonly used by kidney patients include psyllium husk, methylcellulose, and other soluble fiber options. These supplements can help increase fiber intake and support digestive health. It's important to follow the recommended dosage and drink plenty of fluids when taking fiber supplements to prevent potential issues such as intestinal blockages or discomfort.

However, it's crucial to remember that whole foods should be the primary source of fiber in your diet. Fiber supplements should be viewed as a complement to a well-rounded, fiber-rich eating plan.

BALANCING FIBER INTAKE WITH OTHER DIETARY CONSIDERATIONS

When incorporating fiber into your kidney-healthy diet, it's essential to balance fiber intake with other dietary considerations. Here are a few important points to keep in mind:

Fluid Intake: Adequate fluid intake is crucial when consuming a high-fiber diet. Fiber absorbs water, and without sufficient hydration, it may lead to digestive issues such as constipation. Be sure to drink plenty of fluids throughout the day, following your healthcare team's recommendations.

Phosphorus and Potassium: While many high-fiber foods are kidney-friendly, some may also contain higher levels of phosphorus or potassium. If you have specific limitations on these minerals due to your kidney health, it's important to work closely with your healthcare team or registered dietitian to select fiber-rich foods that align with your dietary restrictions.

Individual Tolerance: Every individual's tolerance to fiber varies. Some individuals may need to gradually increase their fiber intake to allow their digestive system to adapt. Pay attention to how your body responds to changes in fiber intake and make adjustments accordingly.

Variety and Balance: Aim for a diverse range of high-fiber foods to ensure you receive a broad spectrum of nutrients. Incorporate fruits, vegetables, whole grains, legumes, and seeds into your meals and snacks. This variety not only enhances the nutritional profile of your diet but also adds culinary enjoyment and promotes overall health.

By including fiber-rich foods, either through whole foods or supplements, you can support your digestive health and overall well-being. Remember to consult with your healthcare team or registered dietitian to tailor your fiber intake to your specific needs and dietary restrictions.

Note: These vegetables have less potassium than other vegetables but if you eat a lot, the amount of potassium can add up. Vegetables are not a significant source of phosphorus.

Food and Serving Size: 1/2 cup cooked, unless stated	Fiber (grams)	Low Potassium (< 100 mg)	Medium Potassium (101 to 200 mg)
Asparagus	2		✓
Broccoli (from frozen)	2		✓
Cabbage	2		✓
Carrots	2		✓
Cauliflower	2	✓	
Cauliflower, cooked from frozen	3		✓
Chayote	2		✓
Corn, yellow	2		✓
Eggplant	2	✓	
Endive, raw	2	✓	
Fuzzy squash (moo qua)	2	✓	
Green beans	2		✓

Green peas, cooked from frozen or canned	4	✓	
Jicama (yambean)	3	✓	
Mushrooms, canned, drained	2		✓
Mushroom, shitake	2	✓	
Pumpkin pie mix, canned (not pure pumpkin)	12		✓
Snap beans, Italian, yellow or green	2		✓
Snow peas	3		✓
Squash, scallop/patty pan	2		✓
Turnip	2		✓
Turnip greens	3		✓
Water chestnuts, canned, drained	2	✓	

| Yardlong beans | 3 | | ✓ |

Note: These fruits have less potassium than other fruits but if you eat a lot, the amount of potassium can add up. Fruit is not a significant source of phosphorus.

Food and Serving Size: 1/2 cup cooked, unless stated	Fiber (grams)	Low Potassium (< 100 mg)	Medium Potassium (101 to 200 mg)
Apple (Medium)	4		✓
Blackberries, fresh or frozen	4		✓
Blueberries, fresh or frozen	2	✓	
Boysenberries, frozen	4	✓	
Cherries	2		✓
Crabapple	2		✓
Cranberries, fresh	2	✓	
Gooseberries, fresh or canned	3		✓
Grapefruit	2		✓
Kumquat, 5	6		✓
Loganberries, frozen	4		✓

Mandarin orange, 1 medium	2		✓
Mango	2		✓
Orange	2		✓
Peach	3		✓
Pear, Asian, 1 medium	4		✓
Pear, canned in syrup, drained	2	✓	
Pear, fresh	3		✓
Prickly pear	3		✓
Prunes, canned in syrup, 5	3		✓
Prunes, stewed, 3	3		✓
Quince	2		✓
Raspberries, fresh	4	✓	
Raspberries, frozen or canned, drained	6		✓
Rhubarb, cooked	3		✓
Strawberries,	2		✓

fresh or frozen			
Tangerine	2		✓

FIBER-RICH CEREALS AND GRAINS

Note: High fiber bread, cereals and grains have more phosphorus and potassium than refined products like white bread.

Food and Serving Size	Fiber (grams)	Low - Medium Potassium < 100 mg	Low - Medium Phosphorus < 70 mg
Breads: 1 slice			
Multi-grain	3	✓	
60% whole wheat	1.5	✓	✓
100% whole wheat	2	✓	
Cereals, Flax, & Bran			
Corn Bran, Quaker ®, 1 cup	6	✓	✓
Frosted Mini Wheat's, Kellogg's®, ½ cup	3	✓	✓
Honey Bunches of Oats, Post, 1	2	✓	

Food			
cup			
Muslix, Kellogg's ®, Apple Crisp, 1/3 cup	2	✓	✓
Shredded Wheat, 1 biscuit	3	✓	
Weetabix, 1 biscuit	2	✓	✓
Oatmeal Quaker ®, quick, minute, large flake, ½ cup cooked	3	high > 100 mg	high > 100 mg
Oatmeal Quaker ®, instant, 1 packet, prepared	3	high > 100 mg	high > 100 mg
Natural Wheat Bran, 2 Tbsp	3	✓	
Grains and Pastas			
Bulgur, ½ cup cooked	3	✓	✓
Barley, ½ cup cooked	2	✓	✓
Pasta, whole wheat, ½ cup cooked	2	✓	✓
Popcorn, popped, no salt, 2 cups	3	✓	✓

| Rice, brown, ½ cup cooked | 2 | ✓ | |
| Rice, wild, ½ cup cooked | 2 | ✓ | |

FIBER-RICH LEGUMES

These foods are high in fiber but they are also high in phosphorous and potassium. Rinse and drain canned beans before using.

Food and Serving Size: ½ cup canned & rinsed or cooked from dry beans*	Fiber (grams)	High Potassium (201-300 mg)	Very High Potassium > 300 mg	High Phosphorus > 100 mg
Baked Beans	7		✓	✓
Black Beans	8		✓	✓
Black-eyed Peas	6	✓		✓
Broad Beans (Fava), canned	6	✓		✓
Broad Beans (Fava)	5		✓	✓
Garbanzo Beans (Chick Peas, Desi, Bengal Gram)	5	✓		✓
Kidney Beans	7		✓	✓
Lentils	5		✓	✓

Lentils (pink/ masoor dal)	4	✓		✓
Lima Beans, canned, mature, white	5	✓		✓
Lima Beans, baby, green, canned or cooked from fresh	5		✓	✓
Navy Beans	7		✓	✓
Pinto Beans	6	✓		✓
Split Peas	3		✓	✓
Soy Beans	6		✓	✓
Soy Beans, Edamame, green	4		✓	✓
White Beans	7		✓	✓

* canned, rinsed legumes are lower in potassium and phosphorus, compared to legumes that are cooked from dry.

FIBER-RICH NUTS AND SEEDS

These foods are high in fiber, but they are also high in phosphorous and potassium.

Food	Serving Size	Fiber (gram	Potassium			Phosphorus		
		am	Low	Medium	High > 200	Low	Medium ium	High gh

		s)	< 100 mg	(100-200 mg)	mg	< 70 mg	(70-100 mg)	> 100 mg
Almonds	15 nuts	2		✓			✓	
Brazil Nuts	6 nuts	2		✓				✓
Chia Seeds	1 Tbsp	4	✓				✓	
Flaxseeds, ground or whole	1 Tbsp	3	✓			✓		
Hazelnuts	15 nuts	2		✓		✓		
Hemp Seeds	2 Tbsp	2		✓				✓
Macadamia nuts	8 nuts	2	✓			✓		
Peanuts	30 nuts	2		✓				✓
Peanut butter	2 Tbsp	2		✓				✓
Pecans	12 nuts	2	✓			✓		
Pistachios	34 nuts	2		✓			✓	

Pumpkin seeds	4 Tbsp	2			✓			✓
Sesame paste	2 Tbsp	2			✓			✓
Sesame seeds	1 Tbsp	2	✓				✓	
Soy nuts	1 Tbsp	2		✓		✓		
Walnut	10 halves	2		✓				✓

You can look up the fiber, potassium and phosphorus content of any food in the USDA FoodData Central (https://fdc.nal.usda.gov/)

CARBS, SUGAR, AND KIDNEY DISEASE

Carbohydrates are a crucial macronutrient that provides energy for the body's daily activities. They are broken down into glucose, which serves as the primary fuel source for cells, including those in the kidneys. Carbohydrates also play a role in maintaining blood glucose levels, supporting brain function, and providing dietary fiber for digestive health.

EXPLORING DIFFERENT TYPES OF CARBS AND THEIR IMPACT ON BLOOD SUGAR LEVELS

When it comes to carbohydrates, not all are created equal. Different types of carbohydrates have varying effects on blood sugar levels. Understanding these differences is crucial for individuals with kidney disease, especially those with diabetes, as it helps in managing blood sugar control effectively. Here are the main types of carbohydrates and their impact on blood sugar levels:

Simple Carbohydrates: Simple carbohydrates consist of one or two sugar molecules and are quickly digested and absorbed by the body. They can cause a rapid spike in blood sugar levels. Examples of simple carbohydrates include table sugar, honey, syrups, and foods made with refined grains (white bread, white rice, and pasta). These foods have little to no fiber or nutritional value. Consuming excessive amounts of simple carbohydrates can lead to unstable blood sugar levels and may increase the risk of complications in individuals with diabetes and kidney disease.

Complex Carbohydrates: Complex carbohydrates are made up of multiple sugar molecules and are digested more slowly than simple carbohydrates. They provide a gradual and sustained release of glucose into the bloodstream, resulting in a more controlled rise in blood sugar levels. Complex carbohydrates are typically found in whole grains, legumes, fruits, and vegetables. These foods are rich in fiber, vitamins, minerals, and other beneficial compounds. The fiber content of complex carbohydrates slows down digestion, promotes satiety, and helps regulate blood sugar levels.

Dietary Fiber: Dietary fiber, which we discussed in the previous chapter, is a type of complex carbohydrate that is indigestible by the human body. It passes through the digestive system relatively intact, adding bulk to the stool and promoting healthy bowel movements. Dietary fiber has minimal impact on blood sugar levels and can even help regulate them. High-fiber foods, such as whole grains, legumes, fruits, vegetables, and nuts, should be emphasized in a kidney-friendly diet. However, it's important to note that not all high-fiber foods are suitable for individuals with advanced kidney disease, as some may contain higher amounts of phosphorus or potassium.

Glycemic Index (GI): The glycemic index is a measure of how quickly a carbohydrate-containing food raises blood sugar levels. Foods with a high glycemic index (GI) are rapidly digested and cause a more significant increase in blood sugar, while foods with a low GI are digested more slowly and have a more gradual impact on blood sugar levels. Choosing low or moderate GI foods can help individuals with kidney disease and diabetes better manage their blood sugar levels. Whole grains, legumes, and non-starchy vegetables generally have a lower GI compared to refined grains and sugary foods.

CARBOHYDRATE RECOMMENDATIONS FOR INDIVIDUALS WITH KIDNEY DISEASE

When it comes to carbohydrate intake, individuals with kidney disease should consider several factors, such as their stage of kidney disease, diabetes management, blood sugar control, and overall nutritional needs. Here are some key recommendations for carbohydrate intake for individuals with kidney disease:

Individualized Approach: Carbohydrate recommendations should be individualized based on factors such as kidney function, diabetes status, medications, and overall health. Working with a registered dietitian who specializes in kidney disease can help determine the appropriate carbohydrate intake for each person's unique needs and health goals.

Blood Sugar Control: For individuals with kidney disease and diabetes, maintaining stable blood sugar levels is essential. Balancing carbohydrate intake with medications, physical activity, and other lifestyle factors is crucial for optimal blood sugar control. It is recommended to monitor blood sugar levels regularly and work with healthcare professionals to adjust medication dosages and timing if needed.

Complex Carbohydrates: Emphasize the consumption of complex carbohydrates that are rich in fiber, vitamins, minerals, and other beneficial compounds. Examples of kidney-friendly complex carbohydrates include whole grains (brown rice, whole wheat bread, quinoa), legumes (beans, lentils), fruits, and non-starchy vegetables. These foods provide sustained energy, promote satiety, and contribute to overall nutritional well-being.

Portion Control: While complex carbohydrates are generally considered healthier options, portion control is still essential. Controlling portion sizes helps manage blood sugar levels and prevents excessive calorie intake. Working with a registered dietitian can provide guidance on appropriate portion sizes and help develop individualized meal plans that meet carbohydrate and overall nutritional goals.

Glycemic Index: Consider the glycemic index (GI) of carbohydrate-containing foods. Foods with a lower GI are digested more slowly, resulting in a slower and more controlled rise in blood sugar levels. Choosing low or moderate GI foods, such as whole grains, legumes, and non-starchy vegetables, can help individuals with kidney disease manage their blood sugar levels effectively.

Monitoring Phosphorus and Potassium Intake: For individuals with advanced kidney disease, it's important to be mindful of the phosphorus and potassium content of carbohydrate-rich foods. Some high-fiber foods, such as whole grains and legumes, may also contain higher levels of phosphorus or potassium, which may need to be limited based on individual dietary restrictions. Consulting with a renal dietitian can help identify suitable carbohydrate sources while managing phosphorus and potassium intake.

Avoiding Added Sugars: Minimize or avoid foods and beverages that contain added sugars, such as sugary drinks, candies, pastries, and sweetened cereals. These sources of simple carbohydrates can lead to rapid spikes in blood sugar levels and provide little nutritional value.

Avoid Artificial Sweeteners: Avoiding artificial sweeteners is a wise choice when it comes to promoting kidney health and overall well-being. Recent studies have shed light on the potential negative impacts of artificial sweeteners on various aspects of our health, including kidney health, heart health, gut health, and more. In a study published in Nature Medicine in February 2023, researchers found a concerning association between the consumption of erythritol, a calorie-free sweetener found in some stevia blends and low-sugar products, and an increased risk for blood clots, heart attacks, and strokes (Witkowski, M., Nemet, I., Alamri, H. *et al.* The artificial sweetener erythritol and cardiovascular event risk. *Nat Med* **29**, 710–718 (2023). https://doi.org/10.1038/s41591-023-02223-9). These findings highlight the importance of being mindful of the potential risks posed by artificial sweeteners and considering healthier alternatives for sweetness in our diet.

TIPS FOR INCORPORATING HEALTHY CARBS INTO A KIDNEY-FRIENDLY DIET

Choose Whole Grains: Opt for whole grain options whenever possible. Whole grains, such as brown rice, whole wheat bread, quinoa, and oats, are rich in fiber, vitamins, and minerals. They provide a steady release of energy, promote satiety, and help maintain stable blood sugar levels.

Include Legumes: Legumes, including beans, lentils, and chickpeas, are excellent sources of complex carbohydrates, fiber, and plant-based protein. They are low in fat and have a low glycemic index, making them suitable for individuals with kidney disease. Legumes can be added to soups, salads, stews, or made into dips like hummus.

Prioritize Non-Starchy Vegetables: Non-starchy vegetables, such as broccoli, spinach, cauliflower, peppers, and cucumbers, are low in carbohydrates and calories while being packed with essential nutrients and fiber. They can be incorporated into meals in various ways, including salads, stir-fries, and roasted vegetable dishes.

Mindful Fruit Selection: Fruits are a natural source of carbohydrates, fiber, vitamins, and minerals. While they are generally considered healthy, some fruits may be higher in potassium or phosphorus. It's important to choose fruits that align with individual dietary restrictions. Opt for lower potassium options such as apples, berries, cherries, and grapes, and limit higher potassium fruits like bananas, oranges, and melons.

Portion Control: Even when consuming healthy carbs, portion control is crucial. Be mindful of the portion sizes to prevent excessive calorie and carbohydrate intake. Working with a registered dietitian can provide guidance on appropriate portion sizes and help create personalized meal plans that meet carbohydrate and overall nutritional goals.

Balance with Protein and Healthy Fats: Pairing healthy carbs with lean protein sources and healthy fats can help create a balanced meal. Protein and fats slow down digestion and promote satiety, which can help manage blood sugar levels and control appetite. Opt for lean sources of protein, such as skinless poultry, fish, tofu, and eggs, and incorporate healthy fats from sources like avocado, nuts, seeds, and olive oil.

Limit Added Sugars: Minimize or avoid foods and beverages with added sugars. Added sugars provide empty calories and can lead to blood sugar spikes. Choose naturally sweet options like fresh fruit or opt for sugar-free alternatives when needed.

Read Food Labels: When purchasing packaged foods, read the nutrition labels carefully. Look for products that are lower in added sugars and high in fiber. Aim for products with whole grains listed as the first ingredient and avoid those that contain refined flours or added sugars.

Meal Planning and Preparation: Plan your meals and snacks in advance to ensure you incorporate healthy carbs throughout the day. By planning, you can make mindful choices and have kidney-friendly options readily available. Consider batch cooking or meal prepping to save time and ensure you have balanced meals on hand.

Work with a Registered Dietitian: Consulting with a registered dietitian who specializes in kidney disease can provide personalized guidance and support in incorporating healthy carbs into your kidney-friendly diet. They can help create a meal plan that aligns with your specific dietary needs, manage blood sugar levels, and optimize overall nutrition.

MANAGING CARBOHYDRATE INTAKE FOR BLOOD SUGAR CONTROL

For individuals with diabetes and kidney disease, monitoring blood sugar levels is crucial. Carbohydrate counting can be a helpful tool to manage blood sugar effectively. It involves keeping track of the total grams of carbohydrates consumed per meal or snack and matching it with an appropriate dose of insulin or diabetes medication. Working with a registered dietitian who specializes in renal nutrition can provide valuable guidance on carbohydrate counting and blood sugar management.

THE IMPACT OF CARBOHYDRATES ON WEIGHT MANAGEMENT

Weight management is often an important aspect of kidney disease management. Carbohydrates can contribute to weight gain if consumed in excess. However, it is essential to note that a well-balanced diet should include carbohydrates for energy and overall nutrition. The key lies in portion control and choosing nutrient-dense carbohydrate sources. By focusing on whole grains, fruits, vegetables, and legumes, individuals can maintain a healthy weight while enjoying the benefits of carbohydrates in their diet.

CALORIES AND KIDNEY HEALTH: BALANCING ENERGY FOR OPTIMAL WELL-BEING

In the journey of managing kidney disease, one often encounters the vital concept of calorie balance. The intricate relationship between calorie intake, weight management, and overall kidney health plays a crucial role in optimizing well-being. In this chapter, we will delve into the intricate details of calories and their impact on kidney health. By understanding the importance of calorie balance, exploring the relationship between calorie intake and weight management, discussing calorie recommendations for individuals with kidney disease, and providing practical tips for monitoring and adjusting calorie intake, we can gain valuable insights into the critical role that calories play in our journey towards improved kidney health.

UNDERSTANDING THE IMPORTANCE OF CALORIE BALANCE IN MANAGING KIDNEY DISEASE

Maintaining a proper calorie balance is crucial for individuals with kidney disease as it directly affects their overall health and well-being. Calorie balance refers to the equilibrium between the calories consumed through food and beverages and the calories expended through physical activity and bodily functions. Here, we will delve deeper into the significance of calorie balance and how it plays a pivotal role in managing kidney disease.

Supporting Energy Levels: Calories serve as the body's primary source of energy. Adequate calorie intake is necessary to fuel the body's daily functions, including physical activity, digestion, and organ function. When the body doesn't receive enough calories, it may lead to feelings of fatigue, weakness, and decreased energy levels. Conversely, excessive calorie intake can result in weight gain, which can strain the kidneys and exacerbate existing health conditions.

Managing Weight: Calorie balance is closely linked to weight management. Achieving and maintaining a healthy weight is crucial for individuals with kidney disease as excess weight can put additional strain on the kidneys. Weight management can help improve kidney function, reduce the risk of complications, and enhance overall health outcomes. By consuming an appropriate number of calories based on individual needs and activity levels, individuals can work towards achieving and maintaining a healthy weight range. Stress, travel, and a busy lifestyle can often disrupt established routines, making it more difficult to maintain a consistent calorie intake. In times of stress, it is common to resort to emotional eating or rely on convenient, calorie-dense foods that may not align with a kidney-friendly diet. Similarly, travel and hectic schedules can lead to limited food options and a temptation to choose calorie-rich, processed foods that may be readily available but lacking in nutritional value. This is one area where I have found it difficult to stay on track.

Promoting Nutritional Adequacy: Calorie balance is intricately tied to achieving a well-rounded and nutritious diet. When individuals consume an appropriate number of calories, they have the opportunity to ensure their meals include a variety of nutrient-dense foods. This allows for a greater intake of essential vitamins, minerals, fiber, and other beneficial compounds that support overall health and help prevent nutrient deficiencies. A balanced and nutrient-rich diet is vital for managing kidney disease and promoting optimal well-being.

Controlling Blood Sugar Levels: For individuals with kidney disease, maintaining stable blood sugar levels is crucial. Calorie balance plays a significant role in managing blood sugar levels, especially for those with diabetes or prediabetes. Consistently consuming an appropriate number of calories throughout the day helps prevent spikes or drops in blood sugar levels, promoting better glucose control. This is particularly important for individuals with both kidney disease and diabetes, as managing blood sugar levels effectively can help slow the progression of kidney damage.

Enhancing Overall Health Outcomes: By achieving a proper calorie balance, individuals with kidney disease can enhance their overall health outcomes. A balanced and controlled calorie intake, combined with a nutrient-rich diet, can support the body's natural healing processes, improve immune function, and reduce the risk of complications associated with kidney disease. By prioritizing calorie balance as part of a comprehensive treatment plan, individuals can take proactive steps towards improving their kidney health and overall well-being.

*DISCUSSING CALORIE RECOMMENDATIONS FOR INDIVIDUALS
WITH KIDNEY DISEASE*

Calorie recommendations for individuals with kidney disease can vary based on several factors, including age, sex, body weight, activity level, and the stage of kidney disease. The goal is to strike a balance that supports overall health, manages weight, and reduces the burden on the kidneys. It is essential to work closely with a registered dietitian who specializes in renal nutrition to determine the appropriate calorie intake for your specific needs. They can consider your individual circumstances and create a personalized plan that aligns with your goals and the stage of your kidney disease.

In general, calorie recommendations for individuals with kidney disease aim to maintain a healthy weight or achieve weight loss if necessary, without compromising nutritional needs. Excess weight can put additional strain on the kidneys and contribute to the progression of kidney disease. On the other hand, unintended weight loss can lead to muscle wasting and nutritional deficiencies. The registered dietitian will assess your body weight and composition, evaluate your nutritional status, and make recommendations accordingly.

The calorie range for individuals with kidney disease typically aligns with standard guidelines for healthy weight management. The range can vary from around 1,500 to 2,500 calories per day for most adults. However, it is crucial to note that these values are approximate, and individual needs may differ.

To determine the appropriate calorie intake, the dietitian will consider factors such as your basal metabolic rate (BMR), which represents the number of calories needed to sustain basic bodily functions at rest, as well as your level of physical activity. They may use equations or specialized tools to estimate your calorie needs accurately.

For individuals with advanced kidney disease or those on dialysis, the dietitian may need to make further adjustments to account for the specific challenges and metabolic changes associated with the condition. In these cases, the focus may be on maintaining adequate nutrient intake while managing fluid and electrolyte balance.

It is important to remember that calorie recommendations should be individualized and regularly reviewed and adjusted based on ongoing assessments and changes in your health status. As kidney function changes or other factors such as weight, physical activity level, or medications evolve, calorie needs may need to be modified accordingly.

Working closely with a registered dietitian will ensure that your calorie recommendations are tailored to your unique needs, taking into account any specific challenges you may face, such as managing fluid intake, sodium restriction, or dietary protein requirements. The dietitian can guide you in creating a meal plan that strikes the right balance of nutrients and calories to support your overall health and kidney function.

Remember, the focus is not solely on calories but also on the quality of the calories you consume. Prioritizing nutrient-dense foods that provide essential vitamins, minerals, and antioxidants is crucial. This means emphasizing whole grains, lean proteins, healthy fats, and a variety of fruits and vegetables. These choices not only contribute to meeting your calorie needs but also support overall health and well-being.

Monitoring and adjusting calorie intake based on individual needs is an essential aspect of managing kidney disease and maintaining overall health. Here are some tips to help you navigate this process:

Work with a Registered Dietitian (You knew this was going to be #1): A registered dietitian who specializes in renal nutrition can provide expert guidance and support in monitoring and adjusting your calorie intake. They will consider your specific needs, medical history, and lifestyle to develop a personalized plan.

Keep a Food Diary: Keeping a detailed record of your daily food intake can be helpful in monitoring calorie intake. Include information about portion sizes, cooking methods, and any added ingredients. A food diary can help you identify patterns, track your progress, and make necessary adjustments.

Use a Food Tracking App: Consider using a food tracking app or website that provides nutrition information for a wide range of foods. These tools can help you monitor your calorie intake more accurately and make informed decisions about your meals and snacks. I personally use Cronometer. It offers a very good free service, but I recommend going with their paid tier that offers even more features (including a web enabled report your healthcare team will love). You can learn more about Cronometer at http://Go.DadviceTV.com/app

Portion Control: Pay attention to portion sizes and practice portion control to manage your calorie intake. Use measuring cups, a food scale, or visual cues to ensure you are consuming appropriate portions. A registered dietitian can provide guidance on portion sizes specific to your needs.

Regular Weigh-ins: Regularly weighing yourself can help you track changes in body weight and adjust your calorie intake accordingly. However, keep in mind that weight alone is not the sole indicator of health. Consult with your healthcare team to determine the appropriate frequency of weigh-ins and the target range for your weight.

Be Mindful of Energy Balance: Energy balance refers to the relationship between calorie intake and expenditure. To maintain a healthy weight, it is important to strike a balance between the calories you consume and the calories you burn through physical activity and bodily functions. If weight loss is a goal, you may need to create a calorie deficit by reducing your intake or increasing your physical activity level.

Adjust Based on Goals and Progress: Regularly assess your progress and consult with your healthcare team to determine if adjustments to your calorie intake are necessary. Depending on your goals and specific needs, you may need to increase or decrease your calorie intake to support weight management, improve nutritional status, or address specific health concerns.

Consider Lifestyle Factors: Take into account lifestyle factors that can impact your calorie needs, such as physical activity level, stress levels, travel, and other daily activities. Discuss these factors with your registered dietitian to ensure that your calorie intake is appropriate for your unique circumstances.

Seek Support and Accountability: Enlist the support of

your healthcare team, family, or friends to help you stay accountable to your calorie monitoring and adjustment goals. Having a support system can provide motivation, encouragement, and guidance throughout your journey.

Remember, the goal is to find the right balance of calories to support your kidney health, manage your weight, and meet your individual needs. Working closely with a registered dietitian will ensure that you receive personalized recommendations and ongoing support in monitoring and adjusting your calorie intake based on your unique circumstances.

DECODING FOOD LABELS: YOUR ROADMAP TO HEALTHY CHOICES

Have you ever wondered what's really in the food you eat? Reading food labels is like unlocking a hidden treasure trove of information that empowers you to make smart and healthy choices. It's your secret weapon for understanding what's inside that package and how it can impact your body and kidney health. By taking a moment to decode those labels, you become an informed shopper, armed with the knowledge to make choices that align with your well-being.

Food labels are like little cheat sheets that spill the beans on what's really in that box or bag. They're your personal detective, revealing the nutritional content and ingredients that lurk within. The Nutrition Facts panel is your best friend, showing you the lowdown on calories, carbs, protein, and fats. It's like a roadmap to help you navigate the nutrient landscape and make choices that fit your dietary needs. And don't forget the ingredient list—it's like a backstage pass that gives you a glimpse into the food's true nature. You can spot potential allergens, sneaky additives, and unhealthy fats hiding in plain sight. Armed with this knowledge, you can make conscious decisions and take control of your kidney health.

Remember, reading food labels is like having a secret superpower. It's a skill that you can develop and use to your advantage. So, grab that magnifying glass and get ready to unravel the mysteries hidden in those labels. Together, we'll embark on a journey of discovery, empowering you to make choices that nourish your body, support your kidney health, and put you on the path to thriving with CKD.

Nutrition Facts	
8 servings per container	
Serving size	**2/3 cup (55g)**
Amount per serving	
Calories	**230**
	% Daily Value*
Total Fat 8g	**10%**
Saturated Fat 1g	**5%**
Trans Fat 0g	
Cholesterol 0mg	**0%**
Sodium 160mg	**7%**
Total Carbohydrate 37g	**13%**
Dietary Fiber 4g	**14%**
Total Sugars 12g	
Includes 10g Added Sugars	**20%**
Protein 3g	
Vitamin D 2mcg	10%
Calcium 260mg	20%
Iron 8mg	45%
Potassium 240mg	6%

* The % Daily Value (DV) tells you how much a nutrient in a serving of food contributes to a daily diet. 2,000 calories a day is used for general nutrition advice.

DECODING SERVING SIZES: THE SIGNIFICANCE IN INTERPRETING NUTRITIONAL INFORMATION

Serving sizes are like the foundation upon which accurate nutrition assessment is built. They provide a standardized measurement that allows you to compare the nutritional content of different foods and make informed choices. However, it's important to be aware that serving sizes can vary significantly and sometimes do not reflect the portions we actually consume. Some manufacturers may manipulate serving sizes to make their products appear healthier than they truly are. This sneaky tactic can lead to confusion and misinterpretation of the nutrient content. By understanding the true significance of serving sizes and learning how to compare them to your own portion sizes, you can navigate this maze and make accurate assessments of your nutrient intake.

Bridging the Gap: Tips for Comparing Serving Sizes to Portion Sizes

Let's face it, we often don't eat the exact amount listed as a serving size on the package. Our portion sizes can vary depending on our hunger, preferences, and circumstances. To accurately assess your nutrient intake, it's crucial to bridge the gap between serving sizes and portion sizes. Here are some tips to help you make meaningful comparisons:

Be Mindful of Portion Distortion: It's easy to lose track of portion sizes, especially when dining out or indulging in our favorite foods. Keep an eye out for portion distortion and be mindful of how much you're actually consuming.

Use Visual Cues: Familiarize yourself with visual cues that can help estimate portion sizes. For example, a serving of meat is roughly the size of a deck of cards, and a serving of pasta is about the size of your fist.

Use Measuring Tools: For more accurate measurements, consider using measuring cups, spoons, or a food scale to portion out your foods. This can provide valuable insights into your nutrient intake and help you make informed choices.

Compare Total Nutrient Content: When comparing products, focus on the total nutrient content rather than relying solely on serving sizes. Pay attention to calories, macronutrients (carbs, protein, fat), sodium, and other relevant nutrients to get a clearer picture of what you're consuming.

UNLOCKING THE NUTRITION FACTS PANEL: BREAKING DOWN THE KEY COMPONENTS

The Nutrition Facts panel is your gateway to understanding the nutritional content of a food product. By decoding its key components, you can make more informed choices:

Serving Size: Pay attention to the serving size, as it dictates the quantities used to determine the nutritional information. Be aware that some manufacturers manipulate serving sizes to make their products seem healthier than they are. Compare the serving size to your typical portion size to accurately assess the nutrient content.

Calories: The calorie count indicates the amount of energy provided by a serving of the food. Understanding the calorie content is crucial for managing weight and maintaining overall health. Consider your daily caloric needs and goals when evaluating the calorie content of a product.

Macronutrients: The panel provides information on carbohydrates, proteins, and fats, which are macronutrients essential for your body's functioning:

- **Carbohydrates**: Carbs provide energy, but not all carbs are created equal. Look for foods with a balance of complex carbohydrates (such as whole grains and vegetables) and limit simple sugars and refined carbs.

- **Proteins**: Proteins are the building blocks of tissues and play a vital role in various bodily functions. Opt for lean protein sources like poultry, fish, legumes, and tofu.

- **Fats**: Fats are necessary for hormone production, insulation, and nutrient absorption. Choose healthier fats like unsaturated fats found in avocados, nuts, and olive oil, while limiting saturated and trans fats.

Fiber: Fiber promotes digestion, helps control blood sugar levels, and supports heart health. Look for foods rich in dietary fiber, such as fruits, vegetables, whole grains, and legumes.

Sugars: Pay attention to the sugar content and distinguish between naturally occurring sugars and added sugars. Added sugars should be limited, as excessive consumption can contribute to various health issues.

Potassium, Calcium, Vitamin D, Iron, and Optional Phosphorus: Additionally, keep an eye out for key nutrients like potassium, calcium, vitamin D, iron, and, optionally, phosphorus. These nutrients play crucial roles in overall health and are particularly important for individuals with kidney disease.

Unveiling Potential Allergens and Common Additives

The Nutrition Facts panel can also help you identify potential allergens and common additives:

Allergens: Manufacturers are required to list common allergens, such as nuts, dairy, soy, wheat, and shellfish, on the label. This information is crucial for individuals with allergies or sensitivities.

Additives: Take note of additives like preservatives, artificial colors, and flavor enhancers. If you prefer to avoid certain additives or have specific dietary restrictions, careful examination of the label can guide your choices.

Assessing Sodium Content

Sodium plays a crucial role in our diet, but excessive intake can have detrimental effects on kidney health. As someone managing kidney disease, monitoring and controlling sodium intake becomes paramount. Sodium has the potential to trigger high blood pressure and accelerate kidney damage, which is why it is the **primary factor** I consider when selecting food products. By understanding how to identify and manage sodium content, we can make informed choices that support our kidney health journey.

Tips for Identifying Hidden Sources of Sodium on Food Labels

Read the Ingredients List: Look for sodium-related terms such as salt, sodium chloride, monosodium glutamate (MSG), sodium bicarbonate, sodium nitrate, or any other ingredient with "sodium" in its name. Be aware that even if a food label does not list "salt" as an ingredient, it may still contain sodium in other forms.

Check the Nutrition Facts Panel: Pay attention to the "Sodium" section, which lists the amount of sodium per serving. Compare this value to your daily sodium target as advised by your healthcare provider. Keep in mind that the serving size might differ from your actual portion size, so adjust the sodium content accordingly.

Watch Out for Hidden Sodium: Some food products, especially processed and packaged items, contain hidden sources of sodium. These can include preservatives, flavor enhancers, and additives. Be cautious of condiments, sauces, salad dressings, canned soups, and processed meats, as they tend to be high in sodium.

Be Mindful of Sodium Claims: Food manufacturers may use phrases like "low-sodium," "reduced sodium," or "no added salt" to promote their products. While these claims can be helpful, it is still essential to review the nutrition facts to ensure the sodium content aligns with your dietary needs.

Choose Fresh and Whole Foods: Opting for fresh fruits, vegetables, and whole grains allows you to have more control over your sodium intake. These natural foods are typically lower in sodium compared to processed alternatives. Incorporate them into your meals and snacks to increase your nutrient intake while minimizing sodium content.

Cook at Home: Preparing your meals from scratch gives you full control over the ingredients and allows you to reduce sodium levels by using alternatives like herbs, spices, and flavorings without added sodium. Experiment with different seasoning blends to enhance the taste of your dishes without relying on excessive salt.

Spotting Hidden Sugars

When it comes to managing kidney disease and maintaining overall health, being aware of hidden sugars in food products is essential. Added sugars not only contribute to weight gain and increase the risk of developing chronic conditions like diabetes and heart disease but can also have a negative impact on kidney health. Understanding how to spot hidden sugars and make informed choices is crucial in supporting your kidney-friendly diet.

Insight into the Various Names and Forms of Added Sugars

Added sugars can go by many names, and food manufacturers often use different forms of sugars to enhance flavor. Some common names and forms of added sugars you may encounter on food labels include:

- Sucrose
- High fructose corn syrup
- Corn syrup
- Dextrose
- Fructose
- Maltose
- Glucose
- Syrup (e.g., rice syrup, maple syrup)
- Molasses
- Honey
- Agave nectar
- Fruit juice concentrates
- Cane sugar
- Brown sugar
- Raw sugar

It's important to note that even seemingly "healthier" alternatives like honey or agave nectar are still sources of added sugars and should be consumed in moderation.

Strategies for Identifying Hidden Sugars in Food Products

Read the Ingredients List: Look for words ending in "-ose" (such as sucrose, fructose, glucose) or any term mentioned in the list above. The higher up on the list, the greater the quantity of added sugar in the product.

Check the Nutrition Facts Panel: Look for the "Total Sugars" section, which includes both naturally occurring and added sugars. Keep in mind that natural sugars found in fruits and dairy products are not a concern. Focus on the "Added Sugars" subcategory to determine the amount of sugars that have been added to the product.

Consider Different Names for Sugar: Besides the obvious terms, added sugars can also be listed as syrups, concentrates, or words that may not be as familiar. Familiarize yourself with the various names used for added sugars to better understand their presence in food products.

Be Wary of Hidden Sugars in Processed Foods: Many processed foods, such as sweetened beverages, flavored yogurt, breakfast cereals, granola bars, and even savory items like condiments and sauces, contain added sugars. Be diligent in reading the labels of these products and choose alternatives with lower sugar content or no added sugars.

Choose Whole Foods: Opting for whole, unprocessed foods like fresh fruits, vegetables, whole grains, and lean proteins can help minimize your exposure to hidden sugars. These foods provide essential nutrients without the added sugars found in processed alternatives.

Be Mindful of "Sugar-Free" Claims: Products labeled as "sugar-free" may not contain traditional sugars, but they can still contain artificial sweeteners. Read the ingredients list to understand what sweeteners are used and whether they are suitable for your dietary preferences and health goals.

EVALUATING INGREDIENT LISTS

When it comes to making informed and healthy choices for your kidney-friendly diet, evaluating ingredient lists plays a crucial role. Ingredient lists provide valuable information about the composition of food products, allowing you to identify potential allergens, avoid harmful additives, and make choices that support your overall health and kidney function.

Guidance on Understanding Ingredient Lists and Their Order of Predominance

The ingredient list is usually found on the packaging of food products and is a valuable tool for understanding what goes into the food you consume. Here are some important points to consider when evaluating ingredient lists:

Order of Predominance: Ingredients are listed in descending order of predominance by weight. The first few ingredients make up the majority of the product, so it's important to pay attention to them. If a specific ingredient you want to limit or avoid appears at the beginning of the list, it may indicate that the product is not suitable for your kidney-friendly diet.

Simplified Names: Some ingredients may have simplified or common names that might not immediately stand out as potentially harmful. For example, sodium bicarbonate is a common ingredient used as a leavening agent in baked goods, but it's also a source of sodium. Being familiar with these simplified names can help you identify ingredients that may impact your kidney health.

Identifying Potential Allergens or Ingredients to Avoid for Individual Dietary Needs

Allergen Labeling: Food products are required to identify common allergens, such as peanuts, tree nuts, soy, milk, eggs, wheat, fish, and shellfish. If you have known allergies or sensitivities, carefully check the ingredient list to avoid any potential triggers.

Phosphorus Additives: Phosphorus is a mineral that individuals with kidney disease often need to monitor. Some food manufacturers may use phosphorus additives in processed foods to enhance texture, taste, or shelf life. Look for ingredients with "PHOS" or "phosphate" in their names, as these additives can contribute to an increased phosphorus load. Remember that phosphorus additives are absorbed by the body at a high rate, and their consumption should be limited to manage phosphorus levels effectively.

Tips for Recognizing Artificial Additives, Preservatives, and Unhealthy Fats

Artificial Additives: Scan the ingredient list for artificial additives such as artificial sweeteners (e.g., aspartame, sucralose), artificial colors (e.g., FD&C Yellow No. 5), or artificial flavors. These additives can be present in various processed foods and may have potential health implications. Opt for foods with minimal artificial additives or choose whole, unprocessed alternatives whenever possible.

Preservatives: Many food products contain preservatives to prolong shelf life. Look out for common preservatives like BHA (butylated hydroxyanisole), BHT (butylated hydroxytoluene), sodium benzoate, or sulfites. While preservatives are generally regarded as safe, some individuals may have sensitivities or prefer to avoid them.

Unhealthy Fats: Check for unhealthy fats, such as trans fats or partially hydrogenated oils. These fats can contribute to inflammation and are generally considered detrimental to heart health. Opt for products with healthier fat sources like monounsaturated fats or polyunsaturated fats.

By carefully evaluating ingredient lists, you can make informed decisions about the foods you consume, ensuring they align with your kidney-friendly diet goals. Pay attention to potential allergens, avoid phosphorus additives when necessary, and be mindful of artificial additives, preservatives, and unhealthy fats.

NAVIGATING HEALTH CLAIMS AND LABELS

When it comes to reading food labels, understanding health claims and labels on food packaging is essential. Food manufacturers often use various claims and labels to promote their products as healthier options. However, it's important to have a critical eye and understand the true significance of these claims. Let's explore some key points to consider when navigating health claims and labels.

Awareness of Common Health Claims on Food Packaging and Their Significance

Low-Fat: This claim suggests that the product contains a reduced amount of fat compared to similar products. However, it's important to note that low-fat doesn't always mean healthy. Some low-fat products compensate for the reduced fat content by adding extra sugar or unhealthy additives. Be sure to evaluate the overall nutritional profile of the product.

Reduced-Sodium: Products with this claim have a lower sodium content compared to their regular counterparts. For individuals with kidney disease, monitoring sodium intake is crucial. However, even reduced-sodium products may still contain significant amounts of sodium. Choose **Low in Sodium** when possible.

Organic: Organic products are grown without the use of synthetic pesticides, genetically modified organisms (GMOs), or artificial additives. While organic labeling is regulated and indicates a specific farming method, it's important to note that organic doesn't automatically mean healthier or superior in terms of nutritional content.

Whole Grain: This claim signifies that the product contains whole grains, which provide more fiber and nutrients compared to refined grains. However, some products labeled as "whole grain" may still contain refined grains as their primary ingredients. Check the ingredient list and ensure whole grains are listed first.

Differentiating Between Terms like "Low-Fat," "Reduced-Sodium," "Organic," etc.

"Low" or "Reduced": These terms indicate that the product contains a lower amount of a specific nutrient compared to a standard or reference product. For example, "low-fat" means the product has a reduced fat content compared to similar products. Pay attention to the actual amounts stated in the

Nutrition Facts panel to understand the significance of the claim.

"Free" or "Zero": These terms suggest that the product contains an insignificant amount of a specific nutrient or ingredient. For instance, "sugar-free" means the product has less than 0.5 grams of sugar per serving. However, be cautious as some "sugar-free" products may contain artificial sweeteners, which might have other health implications.

"Organic": This label indicates that the product meets specific standards for organic production. It ensures that the product is free from synthetic pesticides and other prohibited substances. However, organic doesn't necessarily imply superior nutritional value or absence of unhealthy ingredients.

"Natural": The term "natural" is not well-regulated and can be misleading. It may give the impression of a wholesome and minimally processed product. However, the term "natural" does not have a consistent definition and does not guarantee any specific nutritional benefits.

When evaluating health claims and labels, it's crucial to remember that the most accurate information about the nutritional content and ingredients can be found in the Nutrition Facts panel and the ingredient list. While health claims can be informative, they should be considered alongside the complete picture of the product's nutritional profile.

Navigating the world of food labels may seem overwhelming at first, with all the information and terminology to decipher. However, with practice and a bit of knowledge, you will gradually become adept at spotting foods that align with your dietary needs and preferences. Reading labels becomes an empowering tool in your journey towards a healthier lifestyle.

As you familiarize yourself with label reading, you'll start to notice patterns and become more confident in identifying better food choices. You'll develop a keen eye for ingredients that you want to avoid or limit in your diet, such as excessive sugar, sodium, unhealthy fats, or artificial additives. This knowledge will empower you to make informed decisions that support your overall health and well-being.

One important principle to keep in mind is that the level of processing of a food often correlates with its nutritional value. Generally, heavily processed foods tend to be less favorable choices, as they often contain higher amounts of added sugars, unhealthy fats, and artificial additives. On the other hand, minimally processed or whole foods, such as fruits, vegetables, whole grains, and lean proteins, are typically more nutrient-dense and can be excellent choices for supporting your kidney health.

By gradually understanding the nuances of food labels and recognizing the varying degrees of processing in different products, you will gain confidence in selecting foods that align with your dietary goals. Remember, it's not about perfection or completely eliminating certain foods but making more conscious choices and finding a balance that works for you. With time, reading labels will become second nature, and you'll find yourself easily navigating the aisles of the grocery store, confidently selecting foods that support your kidney health and overall well-being.

FLUID MANAGEMENT: STAYING HYDRATED

In this chapter, we will explore the importance of proper fluid intake in kidney health and discuss strategies for managing fluid intake based on individual needs. We will also provide tips for staying hydrated while considering other dietary restrictions and share ways to make water taste better. Let's dive in and discover how you can effectively stay hydrated for optimal kidney health.

IMPORTANCE OF PROPER FLUID INTAKE IN KIDNEY HEALTH

Maintaining proper fluid balance is vital for kidney health. Adequate hydration supports kidney function by helping to flush out waste products and toxins from the body. It also helps regulate blood pressure and maintain electrolyte balance.

For individuals with kidney disease, proper fluid management becomes even more crucial. Depending on your kidney function and overall health, your healthcare team or registered dietitian will provide specific guidelines on fluid intake to prevent fluid overload or dehydration.

Symptoms of dehydration can vary in severity depending on the degree of fluid loss and individual factors. Here are some common signs and symptoms to watch out for:

- **Increased Thirst**: Feeling excessively thirsty and having a strong desire to drink fluids is one of the first indicators of dehydration.

- **Dry Mouth and Lips**: A dry, sticky feeling in the mouth and lips can be a sign of inadequate fluid intake.

- **Dark-Colored Urine**: When you're dehydrated, your urine becomes more concentrated, resulting in a darker color. In severe dehydration, urine may appear amber or even brown.

- **Decreased Urination**: Reduced frequency of urination or passing very small amounts of urine can be a sign of dehydration.

- **Fatigue and Weakness**: Dehydration can cause feelings of fatigue, weakness, and a lack of energy as the body's cells do not receive adequate hydration.

- **Dizziness or lightheadedness**: Inadequate fluid intake can affect blood pressure and circulation, leading to dizziness or lightheadedness.

- **Headache**: Dehydration can trigger headaches or worsen existing headaches.

- **Dry Skin**: When the body is dehydrated, the skin may feel dry, less elastic, and appear dull.

- **Muscle Cramps**: Insufficient fluid intake can result in muscle cramps, especially during physical activity or in hot environments.

- **Rapid Heartbeat**: Dehydration can lead to an increased heart rate or palpitations.

It's important to note that these symptoms may not be exclusive to dehydration and can be caused by other factors.

If you experience severe or persistent symptoms, it's crucial to seek medical attention and consult with your healthcare provider.

HYDRATION LEVEL AND EGFR

The hydration level of an individual can indeed impact the estimated glomerular filtration rate (eGFR) reported in lab tests. It's important to understand the relationship between hydration and eGFR to interpret these results accurately and avoid potential misinterpretations.

Dehydration, or inadequate fluid intake, can lead to a decrease in blood volume and concentration, which affects the filtration process in the kidneys. When the body is dehydrated, blood flow to the kidneys may decrease, resulting in a temporary decrease in eGFR. As a result, the reported eGFR value may be lower than the actual kidney function.

Conversely, overhydration, or excessive fluid intake, can temporarily increase blood volume and dilute the concentration of waste products in the blood. This can artificially elevate the eGFR value, making it appear higher than the actual kidney function. It's essential to note that artificially elevated eGFR values due to overhydration **do not** reflect improved kidney function.

It's crucial to emphasize that attempting to overhydrate solely to achieve better-looking lab results is not advisable. Artificially manipulating hydration levels can lead to inaccurate interpretations and misguide healthcare decisions. It's far more important to focus on maintaining adequate hydration levels as part of your overall kidney health and general well-being.

Remember, accurate labs serve as valuable tools and a roadmap to guide your healthcare team in providing appropriate care and interventions. Open communication with your healthcare provider, adherence to recommended fluid intake guidelines, and maintaining a healthy lifestyle are the keys to supporting your kidney health and overall well-being.

STRATEGIES FOR MANAGING FLUID INTAKE BASED ON INDIVIDUAL NEEDS

Fluid management is highly individualized, and recommendations may vary depending on your stage of kidney disease, urine output, and any underlying medical conditions. Here are some general strategies for managing fluid intake:

Follow Your Healthcare Team's Recommendations: Your healthcare team will provide personalized guidelines for fluid intake based on your specific needs. It's important to adhere to these recommendations and regularly communicate any changes or concerns.

Monitor Urine Output: Pay attention to your urine output as it can serve as a valuable indicator of your fluid balance. If you notice a significant decrease or increase in urine output, consult with your healthcare team.

Measure Fluids: Keep track of your fluid intake by measuring and recording the amount of fluids consumed throughout the day. This can help you stay within the recommended limits and avoid excessive or insufficient fluid intake.

Spread Fluid Intake: Distribute your fluid intake evenly throughout the day, rather than consuming large amounts at once. This allows for better fluid absorption and helps maintain a more stable fluid balance.

TIPS FOR STAYING HYDRATED WHILE CONSIDERING OTHER DIETARY RESTRICTIONS

Staying hydrated is important, but it's equally crucial to consider any other dietary restrictions you may have. Here are some tips to stay hydrated while managing other dietary concerns:

Limit Fluids with High Sodium or Potassium: If you have specific sodium or potassium restrictions, be mindful of the fluids you consume. Avoid high-sodium beverages such as sodas, sports drinks, or certain fruit juices. Choose low-sodium or sodium-free options whenever possible. Similarly, be cautious of high-potassium drinks like coconut water or certain fruit juices if you have potassium restrictions.

Incorporate Hydrating Foods: In addition to fluids, certain foods can contribute to your overall hydration. Include water-rich foods such as cucumbers, cantaloupe, honeydew melon, lemon, strawberries, cherries, and other fruits and vegetables in your diet. These foods can provide hydration along with essential nutrients.

Manage Fluids with Sugar: While store-bought water flavorings can add variety to your water, be cautious of high sugar content. Opt for sugar-free or low-sugar alternatives. You can enhance the taste of water naturally by adding slices of lemon, cucumber, or berries to your water, which can infuse flavor without adding excessive sugars.

WAYS TO MAKE WATER TASTE BETTER

To make water more enjoyable, you can experiment with different ways to add flavor. Here are some ideas:

True Lemon Water Flavorings: Utilize True Lemon water flavorings, especially the dark cherry and lemon flavors, which can add a refreshing twist to your water. These flavorings offer convenience without the added sugars found in many store-bought water flavorings.

Infuse Water with Fruits and Vegetables: Enhance the taste of water by infusing it with fruits and vegetables. Try adding slices of cucumber, cantaloupe, honeydew melon, lemon, strawberries, or cherries to your water. These natural additions can add subtle flavors and a refreshing touch without compromising your kidney-friendly diet.

Herbal Infusions: Explore herbal infusions by steeping herbs like mint, basil, or lemongrass in water. These herbs can provide a pleasant aroma and a hint of flavor to elevate your hydration experience.

Citrus Zest: Grate some citrus zest, such as lemon or orange, into your water for a burst of citrusy fragrance and taste. This simple addition can make plain water more enjoyable.

Remember to be mindful of the overall sugar content in any flavorings or additives. Moderation is key, and it's important to balance flavor enhancement with your individual dietary needs and restrictions.

By implementing these tips and strategies, you can stay adequately hydrated while considering your specific dietary concerns and preferences. Fluid management plays a vital role in supporting kidney health, and finding ways to make water more enjoyable can encourage you to maintain proper hydration throughout the day.

QUENCHING YOUR THIRST: NAVIGATING BEVERAGES FOR KIDNEY HEALTH

In the quest for optimal kidney health, the beverages we choose play a significant role. In this chapter we will explore the world of kidney-friendly beverages, helping you make informed choices that nourish and support your kidneys. From the best hydrator to the options that should be limited or avoided, let's dive into the realm of beverages for kidney disease.

FINDING KIDNEY-FRIENDLY BEVERAGES

When selecting beverages for a kidney-friendly diet, it's important to consider certain factors, such as sugar content, nutrient composition, and potential impact on kidney function. Here's what to look for in a kidney-friendly beverage:

- Low Sugar Content: Excessive sugar intake can lead to weight gain, diabetes, and other health issues, which can further burden the kidneys. Opt for beverages with low or no added sugars to promote kidney health and overall well-being.

- Hydration: Adequate hydration is essential for kidney

function. Choose beverages that help maintain proper hydration levels without excessive sodium or other additives. Water is the best choice for optimal hydration.

· Nutritional Value: Some beverages offer additional nutrients that can benefit kidney health. Look for options that provide essential vitamins and minerals while being mindful of any specific dietary restrictions or recommendations.

RECOMMENDED BEVERAGES

Water: Water is the ultimate kidney-friendly beverage. It hydrates the body without adding extra calories, sugar, or sodium. Aim to drink plenty of water throughout the day to support optimal kidney function and overall health. The chapter FLUID MANAGEMENT: STAYING HYDRATED has recommendations on how to add flavor to water while staying kidney-friendly.

Clear Sodas: Clear sodas, such as lemon-lime or ginger ale, can be a refreshing choice for kidney-friendly hydration. Look for options with low or no added sugars and avoid those with high phosphorus content. Remember to enjoy them in moderation.

Herbal Teas: Herbal teas, such as chamomile, peppermint, or hibiscus, offer a flavorful and hydrating option without the caffeine found in traditional teas. These caffeine-free options can be enjoyed hot or cold and can provide a pleasant alternative to other beverages.

Coffee: In moderation, coffee can be a kidney-friendly beverage. It provides a boost of energy and may have some antioxidant properties. However, be mindful of your individual tolerance to caffeine and any specific dietary restrictions related to potassium or phosphorus.

Nutritional Drinks: Certain nutritional drinks, like low-phosphorus or low-potassium shakes, can be beneficial for individuals with specific dietary needs. These drinks are formulated to provide essential nutrients while considering the restrictions of a kidney-friendly diet. Consult with a renal dietitian to determine the most suitable options for your individual requirements.

White Milk: White milk can be a good source of protein, calcium, and vitamin D. Choose low-fat or skim milk to minimize saturated fat content. However, be mindful of your individual dietary needs, including protein and phosphorus restrictions. I'll discuss milk and milk alternatives in detail in the next chapter.

Clear Energy Drinks: If you need an energy boost, opt for clear energy drinks that are low in sugar and caffeine. However, it's important to use them sparingly and consult with your healthcare team, as excessive consumption can have negative effects on kidney health.

Low-Sodium Tomato Juice: Tomato juice can be a tasty and hydrating option, but choose low-sodium varieties to reduce sodium intake. Tomatoes are rich in lycopene, an antioxidant that may have potential benefits for kidney health.

BEVERAGES TO LIMIT OR AVOID

Dark Sodas/Colas: Dark sodas and colas tend to contain phosphoric acid, which can contribute to higher phosphorus levels in the body. Limit consumption of these beverages to avoid potential complications for kidney health.

Diet Sodas with Artificial Sweeteners: Although diet sodas are low in sugar, they often contain artificial sweeteners that may have their own health implications. Some studies suggest a potential link between artificial sweeteners and negative effects on kidney function and heart health. It's best to limit or avoid these beverages and opt for other kidney-friendly options instead.

Fruit Juices: Fruit juices can be high in natural sugars and phosphorus. While they may provide some vitamins and minerals, it's important to consume them in moderation and consider their impact on blood sugar levels and phosphorus balance.

Alcoholic Beverages: Alcohol consumption can have a dehydrating effect on the body and may interfere with kidney function. It's essential to limit or avoid alcohol, especially if you have advanced kidney disease or certain medical conditions that contraindicate alcohol consumption.

Chocolate Milk: Chocolate milk is often high in sugar and phosphorus, which can be detrimental to kidney health. Limit consumption of chocolate milk or consider alternatives like low-fat or skim white milk.

PERSONALIZING YOUR BEVERAGE CHOICES

Every individual's dietary needs and preferences may vary. Work closely with your healthcare team, including a renal dietitian, to tailor your beverage choices to your specific requirements. They can provide guidance on portion sizes, recommended brands, and alternatives based on your lab results and overall health condition.

By personalizing your beverage choices and embracing kidney-friendly options, you can nourish your body, support kidney function, and optimize your overall well-being.

Choosing kidney-friendly beverages is an essential component of a balanced and health-conscious diet for individuals with kidney disease. By opting for hydrating, low-sugar options like water, clear sodas, herbal teas, and nutritional drinks, you can support your kidney health while satisfying your thirst. Be mindful of the beverages to limit or avoid, such as dark sodas, diet sodas with artificial sweeteners, fruit juices, alcoholic beverages, and sports drinks.

MILK AND KIDNEY DISEASE: EXPLORING THE RELATIONSHIP

In this chapter, we will delve into the relationship between milk and kidney health. Milk is a widely consumed beverage that provides essential nutrients, but there are various considerations for individuals with kidney disease. We will explore the impact of milk on kidney health, discuss different types of milk and their nutritional content, and address common misconceptions and concerns regarding milk consumption in kidney disease. Understanding the role of milk in a kidney-healthy diet will empower you to make informed choices for your overall well-being.

UNDERSTANDING THE IMPACT OF MILK ON KIDNEY HEALTH

Milk is often associated with essential nutrients like calcium, protein, and vitamin D, making it an important component of a balanced diet. Here, we will delve deeper into the role of milk in providing these vital nutrients and its impact on kidney health.

Essential Nutrients in Milk:

Milk is a rich source of calcium, a mineral that plays a crucial role in maintaining healthy bones and teeth. Adequate calcium intake is particularly important for individuals with kidney disease, as they may be at a higher risk of developing bone-related complications. Protein, another essential nutrient found in milk, is vital for various bodily functions, including tissue repair, immune support, and the production of enzymes and hormones. Additionally, milk contains vitamin D, which aids in the absorption of calcium and contributes to bone health.

Fluid Balance, Electrolytes, and Blood Pressure:

Fluid balance and electrolyte levels are crucial considerations in kidney health. While milk is a fluid, it is important to understand its impact on fluid balance for individuals with kidney disease. Consuming milk can contribute to overall fluid intake and must be monitored in cases where fluid restriction is necessary. Electrolytes like sodium and potassium are also present in milk, and their levels can affect fluid balance and blood pressure. Individuals with kidney disease may need to adjust their milk consumption to align with their specific dietary recommendations.

Role of Milk in Bone Health and Osteoporosis Prevention:

Bone health is a significant concern for individuals with kidney disease, as mineral imbalances and compromised kidney function can weaken bones. Milk's high calcium content makes it a valuable dietary source for promoting bone health. Adequate calcium intake, along with other lifestyle factors, can help reduce the risk of osteoporosis and fractures. Vitamin D, present in milk, aids in calcium absorption, further supporting bone health. It is important to work with your healthcare team or dietitian to determine the appropriate amount of milk and other calcium sources needed to maintain optimal bone health while considering kidney-specific dietary restrictions.

By understanding the role of milk in providing essential nutrients, its potential impact on fluid balance, electrolyte levels, and blood pressure, as well as its contribution to bone health, you can make informed decisions about incorporating milk into your kidney-healthy diet.

EXPLORING DIFFERENT TYPES OF MILK AND THEIR NUTRITIONAL CONTENT

When it comes to choosing milk, there are various options available, including cow's milk, plant-based milk alternatives, and lactose-free milk. Understanding the nutritional composition of different types of milk is essential for individuals with kidney disease, especially those with specific dietary needs or restrictions. Let's delve into the details of these milk options and discuss considerations for individuals with specific dietary requirements.

Cow's Milk:

Cow's milk is a traditional and widely consumed milk variety. It is a rich source of essential nutrients, including protein, calcium, vitamin D, and other vitamins and minerals. The nutritional content of cow's milk can vary depending on factors such as the breed of cow, processing methods, and fat content (whole, reduced-fat, or skim milk). Whole milk has a higher fat content, while reduced-fat and skim milk options contain lower fat levels.

Plant-Based Milk Alternatives:

Plant-based milk alternatives have gained popularity among individuals with dietary restrictions, including those with lactose intolerance or following a vegan lifestyle. These alternatives are typically made from plants such as almonds, soy, oats, rice, or coconut. They offer a range of flavors and textures to suit different preferences. It's important to note that the nutritional composition of plant-based milk alternatives can differ significantly from cow's milk. While they may be lower in protein, they can provide other nutrients such as calcium, vitamin D (if fortified), and certain plant compounds. Reading the labels and choosing fortified options can help ensure an adequate intake of essential nutrients.

Lactose-Free Milk:

For individuals with lactose intolerance, lactose-free milk can be a suitable option. Lactose-free milk is cow's milk that has been treated with the enzyme lactase, which breaks down lactose into simpler forms that are easier to digest. This allows individuals with lactose intolerance to enjoy milk without experiencing digestive discomfort. Lactose-free milk retains the nutritional profile of regular cow's milk, providing similar amounts of protein, calcium, and other nutrients.

CONSIDERATIONS FOR SPECIFIC DIETARY NEEDS

Individuals with specific dietary needs, such as lactose intolerance or allergies, should carefully consider their milk choices. Here are some important points to consider:

Lactose Intolerance: If you are lactose intolerant, opting for lactose-free milk or plant-based milk alternatives can help you avoid discomfort while still obtaining essential nutrients.

Allergies: Individuals with milk allergies should avoid cow's milk and opt for plant-based milk alternatives that do not contain milk proteins. It's important to read labels carefully, as some individuals with milk allergies may also need to avoid certain plant-based milk options that are processed in facilities that handle allergens.

Nutritional Considerations: When selecting a milk type, consider your overall dietary requirements and goals. If you have specific nutritional needs, such as protein requirements, you may need to explore additional protein sources if you opt for plant-based milk alternatives, which generally contain less protein than cow's milk.

DISCUSSING CONSIDERATIONS FOR INCORPORATING MILK IN A KIDNEY-HEALTHY DIET

Incorporating milk into a kidney-healthy diet requires careful consideration, as dietary recommendations for individuals with kidney disease are highly individualized. Several factors, such as the stage of kidney disease, protein restrictions, and fluid balance, need to be taken into account when determining the appropriate role of milk in a kidney-healthy meal plan. Let's explore these considerations in more detail and provide practical tips for incorporating milk while considering other dietary restrictions.

Individualized Nature of Dietary Recommendations:

It is important to recognize that dietary recommendations for kidney disease management are highly individualized. The guidelines and restrictions vary depending on factors such as the stage of kidney disease, level of kidney function, presence of other health conditions, and individual nutritional needs. Therefore, it is crucial to consult with your healthcare team or registered dietitian to receive personalized guidance that aligns with your specific dietary requirements.

Guidelines for Milk Consumption:

The guidelines for milk consumption in kidney disease management can vary based on individual factors. Here are some considerations:

Stage of Kidney Disease: The recommendations for milk consumption may differ based on the stage of kidney disease. In early stages, milk can be included as a source of essential nutrients. However, as kidney function declines, modifications to milk intake may be necessary to manage fluid balance, protein restrictions, and other nutritional needs.

Protein Restrictions: Individuals with advanced kidney disease may have protein restrictions to manage the buildup of waste products in the body. In such cases, it is important to consider the protein content of milk and balance it with other protein sources to meet individual dietary goals.

Fluid Balance: Fluid intake is an important consideration in kidney disease management, as excessive fluid intake can strain the kidneys. Milk is a fluid, and its consumption must be monitored in cases where fluid restriction is necessary.

Practical Tips for Incorporating Milk:

Here are some practical tips for incorporating milk into a kidney-healthy meal plan while considering other dietary restrictions:

Portion Control: Pay attention to portion sizes when consuming milk to manage protein and fluid intake. Your healthcare team or dietitian can provide guidance on the appropriate serving size based on your individual needs.

Balance with Other Nutrients: Consider the overall nutritional composition of your meals and balance the intake of other nutrients alongside milk. This includes considering sources of protein, carbohydrates, and fats to ensure a well-rounded meal plan.

Personalized Meal Planning: Work with your healthcare team or registered dietitian to develop a personalized meal plan that incorporates milk while considering other dietary restrictions and individual nutritional needs. They can help you create a balanced diet that aligns with your specific goals and supports kidney health.

COMMON MISCONCEPTIONS AND CONCERNS REGARDING MILK

Misconceptions and concerns surrounding milk consumption in kidney disease can lead to confusion and unnecessary dietary restrictions. It is important to address these misconceptions and provide evidence-based insights to help individuals make informed decisions about including milk in their diet. Let's address some common misconceptions and concerns and provide clarity based on scientific evidence.

Avoiding Milk Completely:

One common misconception is that all individuals with kidney disease should avoid milk completely. However, this is not necessarily true. The suitability of milk in a kidney-healthy diet depends on individual factors such as the stage of kidney disease, protein restrictions, and fluid balance. It is important to consult with your healthcare team or registered dietitian to determine the appropriate role of milk in your specific dietary plan.

Impact on Kidney Function:

There is a concern that milk consumption may negatively impact kidney function. However, scientific research suggests that moderate milk consumption is generally well-tolerated and does not harm kidney function in individuals with normal kidney function or early stages of kidney disease. In fact, milk can provide important nutrients such as calcium, protein, and vitamin D, which are beneficial for overall health.

Calcium and Kidney Stones:

Some individuals worry that milk, which is a source of calcium, may contribute to the formation of kidney stones. However, studies have shown that dietary calcium from milk is not associated with an increased risk of kidney stones. In fact, adequate calcium intake may help reduce the risk of certain types of kidney stones. It is important to note that individualized recommendations may be necessary based on the type of kidney stones and other factors, and consulting with a healthcare professional or registered dietitian is crucial.

Lactose Intolerance and Allergies:

Individuals with lactose intolerance or allergies may have concerns about consuming milk. However, there are alternatives available, such as lactose-free milk or plant-based milk options, that can be considered. These alternatives can provide similar nutritional benefits while addressing specific dietary needs and preferences.

Personalized Approach:

It is important to emphasize that dietary recommendations for individuals with kidney disease should be personalized. The impact of milk consumption can vary depending on individual factors such as the stage of kidney disease, protein restrictions, and fluid balance. Consulting with a healthcare professional or registered dietitian is essential to receive personalized guidance that aligns with your specific dietary requirements.

THE DANGERS OF STAR FRUIT (CARAMBOLA) AND KIDNEY DISEASE

Star fruit, also known as carambola, with its vibrant appearance and unique taste, may seem like an enticing addition to a fruit-loving individual's diet. However, for individuals with kidney disease, star fruit poses a significant health risk. This chapter aims to shed light on the dangers of star fruit (carambola) and its potential toxic effects on kidney function. By understanding these risks, individuals with kidney disease can make informed decisions to protect their kidney health.

HIGHLIGHTING THE UNIQUE RISKS ASSOCIATED WITH STAR FRUIT

Star fruit, also known as carambola, may be visually appealing and have a distinct flavor, but it harbors unique risks for individuals with kidney disease. Unlike many other fruits, star fruit contains a naturally occurring toxin called oxalate. While the majority of individuals can safely consume star fruit without any adverse effects, for those with compromised kidney function, the oxalate content in star fruit can pose serious health complications. The kidneys play a vital role in filtering toxins from the bloodstream, including the oxalate found in star fruit. However, individuals with kidney disease may experience difficulties in eliminating oxalate, leading to its accumulation in the body and potentially causing harm to the kidneys and other organs. This heightened sensitivity to oxalate makes star fruit a significant concern for individuals with kidney disease, requiring them to exercise caution and avoid its consumption altogether.

DISCUSSING THE TOXIC EFFECTS OF STAR FRUIT ON KIDNEY FUNCTION

Consuming star fruit can have severe consequences on kidney function, particularly for individuals with kidney disease. The unique toxin present in star fruit, called oxalate, can prove highly toxic to the kidneys. When ingested, oxalate can accumulate in the body, overwhelming the kidneys' ability to filter it out effectively. This accumulation can lead to a condition known as star fruit nephrotoxicity, which manifests as kidney damage and impairment.

The toxic effects of star fruit on kidney function extend beyond mere impairment. The oxalate can interfere with normal cellular processes in the kidneys, disrupting their ability to maintain electrolyte balance and regulate fluid levels. This disruption can result in electrolyte imbalances, such as hyperkalemia (high levels of potassium in the blood) or hypercalcemia (high levels of calcium in the blood), which further burden the kidneys and compromise their function.

Moreover, star fruit nephrotoxicity can trigger neurological symptoms, as the oxalate toxin affects the central nervous system. Neurological manifestations may include confusion, mental disorientation, seizures, hiccups, and in severe cases, even coma. These symptoms arise from the build-up of neurotoxic substances in the body due to impaired kidney function caused by star fruit ingestion.

It is important to emphasize that the toxic effects of star fruit on kidney function are not limited to individuals with advanced kidney disease. Even individuals with mild kidney impairment or those at risk of developing kidney disease should exercise caution and avoid consuming star fruit. The potential harm it poses to kidney health makes it imperative to prioritize kidney safety by eliminating star fruit from the diet entirely.

PROVIDING GUIDANCE ON AVOIDING STAR FRUIT AND POTENTIAL ALTERNATIVES

To safeguard kidney health, it is crucial for individuals with kidney disease to completely avoid consuming star fruit. Even a small quantity of star fruit can trigger the toxic effects associated with its oxalate content. Here are some practical steps to steer clear of star fruit and explore alternative fruit choices for a varied and nutritious diet:

Educate yourself: Learn to recognize star fruit and its various forms, including fresh, dried, juice, or as an ingredient in prepared foods or beverages. Read food labels carefully, especially when trying new products or dining out, to ensure star fruit is not present.

Communicate with healthcare professionals: Inform your healthcare team, including your nephrologist and renal dietitian, about the potential risks associated with star fruit and your commitment to avoiding it. Seek their guidance in developing a personalized meal plan that excludes star fruit and aligns with your specific dietary needs.

Explore alternative fruits: While star fruit may be off-limits, there is a wide array of delicious and kidney-friendly fruits to choose from. Some excellent alternatives include apples, berries (such as strawberries, blueberries, or raspberries), grapes, pineapples, peaches, pears, and melons (such as cantaloupe or watermelon). These fruits provide essential vitamins, minerals, and dietary fiber, promoting overall health and supporting kidney function.

Embrace variety: To enhance your fruit selection, rotate and experiment with different options. Try seasonal fruits, explore exotic choices, and diversify your fruit intake to ensure a broad spectrum of nutrients while adding interest to your meals and snacks.

Consult your renal dietitian: Engage with a renal dietitian who can provide personalized guidance on suitable fruit choices based on your specific health needs and stage of kidney disease. They can help tailor a meal plan that ensures optimal nutrition while prioritizing kidney health.

THE ROLE OF GUT HEALTH IN KIDNEY DISEASE

The intricate relationship between gut health and kidney health is an emerging area of scientific research. The gut, also known as the gastrointestinal tract, is home to trillions of microorganisms collectively referred to as the gut microbiota. These microorganisms play a vital role in various aspects of our health, including kidney function. In this chapter, we will delve into the connection between gut health and kidney disease, explore the impact of gut microbiota on kidney function, discuss dietary and lifestyle strategies to support a healthy gut, and highlight the potential benefits of probiotics and prebiotics in kidney disease management.

UNDERSTANDING THE CONNECTION BETWEEN GUT HEALTH AND KIDNEY HEALTH

The connection between gut health and kidney health is a fascinating area of research that is shedding new light on the intricate relationship between these two vital systems in our body. The gut, or gastrointestinal tract, is home to trillions of microorganisms collectively known as the gut microbiota. These microorganisms play a crucial role in various aspects of our health, including the function and well-being of our kidneys.

One key aspect of this connection lies in the immune system. The gut is home to a significant portion of our immune cells, and it serves as the first line of defense against harmful substances and pathogens. A healthy gut microbiota helps to maintain a balanced and regulated immune response, which is important for preventing chronic inflammation. Chronic inflammation is a common factor in the development and progression of kidney disease, as it can contribute to kidney damage and impair kidney function.

Furthermore, the gut microbiota is involved in the metabolism of various substances, including drugs and dietary components. Some gut bacteria have the ability to metabolize certain medications and toxins, influencing their absorption, distribution, and elimination from the body. In the context of kidney health, this can have implications for the processing and excretion of waste products and drugs that can potentially impact kidney function.

Moreover, the gut microbiota produces a range of metabolites, including short-chain fatty acids (SCFAs), which have been shown to have anti-inflammatory, antioxidant, and immune-regulating properties. These metabolites can help maintain a healthy gut environment and support overall kidney health. Additionally, SCFAs have been found to play a role in regulating blood pressure, which is a crucial factor in maintaining kidney health.

Imbalances or dysbiosis in the gut microbiota, characterized by a disruption in the composition and diversity of beneficial and harmful bacteria, have been linked to an increased risk of kidney disease and its progression. Dysbiosis can lead to chronic inflammation, oxidative stress, impaired gut barrier function, and altered immune responses, all of which can impact kidney health.

Understanding the connection between gut health and kidney health emphasizes the importance of maintaining a healthy gut microbiota for optimal kidney function. Strategies that promote a healthy gut, such as consuming a fiber-rich diet, staying hydrated, managing stress levels, and avoiding factors that disrupt the gut microbiota (such as excessive use of antibiotics or a highly processed diet), can contribute to better kidney health.

EXPLORING THE IMPACT OF GUT MICROBIOTA ON KIDNEY FUNCTION

Emerging research suggests that the gut microbiota plays a crucial role in maintaining kidney health and preventing the progression of kidney disease. Healthy gut microbiota helps in the metabolism of various substances, such as dietary nutrients and drugs, which can directly impact kidney function. Additionally, the gut microbiota produces metabolites, such as short-chain fatty acids, that have anti-inflammatory and antioxidant properties, which are beneficial for kidney health. Imbalances or dysbiosis in the gut microbiota, characterized by a decrease in beneficial bacteria and an increase in harmful bacteria, can contribute to the development and progression of kidney disease.

DIETARY AND LIFESTYLE STRATEGIES TO SUPPORT A HEALTHY GUT FOR OPTIMAL KIDNEY HEALTH

Emphasize a plant-based, fiber-rich diet: Consuming a variety of fruits, vegetables, whole grains, legumes, and nuts provides dietary fiber that promotes a healthy gut microbiota. Fiber acts as a prebiotic, nourishing beneficial bacteria in the gut.

Stay adequately hydrated: Drinking enough water helps maintain healthy bowel movements and supports the transport of nutrients to the gut microbiota.

Limit processed foods and added sugars: High consumption of processed foods and added sugars can disrupt the balance of gut microbiota and contribute to inflammation and metabolic disturbances.

Manage stress levels: Chronic stress can impact the gut-brain axis and disrupt the gut microbiota. Engaging in stress-reducing activities such as meditation, yoga, or hobbies can support a healthy gut environment.

HIGHLIGHTING THE POTENTIAL BENEFITS OF PROBIOTICS AND PREBIOTICS

Probiotics are beneficial bacteria that, when consumed in adequate amounts, can confer health benefits. They have shown promise in reducing inflammation, improving gut barrier function, and modulating immune responses, which can positively impact kidney health. Prebiotics, on the other hand, are non-digestible fibers that serve as food for beneficial gut bacteria, promoting their growth and activity. Both probiotics and prebiotics can be beneficial in maintaining a healthy gut microbiota and supporting kidney health.

It is important to note that specific recommendations for probiotic and prebiotic supplementation should be individualized and guided by healthcare professionals, considering the unique needs and health status of each individual.

GETTING MORE IRON: ENHANCING IRON INTAKE FOR KIDNEY HEALTH

In this chapter, we will explore the importance of iron in the kidney diet and discuss strategies to enhance iron intake. We will delve into iron's role in kidney disease and anemia, iron-rich foods, maximizing iron absorption, balancing iron intake with other dietary considerations, and the use of iron supplements. Understanding how to optimize iron intake will contribute to maintaining overall kidney health and managing anemia effectively.

UNDERSTANDING IRON'S ROLE IN KIDNEY DISEASE AND ANEMIA

Iron is an essential mineral that plays a crucial role in various bodily functions, including the production of red blood cells and oxygen transport. In kidney disease, anemia is a common complication that occurs due to reduced production of erythropoietin, a hormone responsible for stimulating red blood cell production. Anemia can lead to symptoms such as fatigue, weakness, shortness of breath, and poor concentration. Adequate iron intake becomes even more critical to support the production of healthy red blood cells.

IRON-RICH FOODS AND STRATEGIES FOR MAXIMIZING IRON ABSORPTION

Incorporating iron-rich foods into your kidney-friendly diet is vital for meeting your iron needs. Here are some kidney-friendly sources of iron:

Lean Meats and Poultry: Animal-based sources of iron, such as lean beef, lamb, pork, and poultry (chicken, turkey), provide heme iron, which is highly bioavailable and easily absorbed by the body. Include small portions of these meats in your diet to boost your iron intake.

Fish and Seafood: Certain types of fish and seafood are excellent sources of iron. Examples include salmon, tuna, mackerel, oysters, clams, and shrimp. Incorporate these nutrient-rich options into your meals to increase your dietary iron.

Legumes and Pulses: Plant-based sources of iron, such as beans, lentils, chickpeas, and tofu, offer a good amount of non-heme iron. While non-heme iron is not as easily absorbed as heme iron, combining these plant-based iron sources with foods rich in vitamin C can enhance iron absorption. Consider pairing legumes with citrus fruits, tomatoes, or bell peppers to optimize iron absorption.

Nuts and Seeds: Certain nuts and seeds are excellent sources of iron. Almonds, cashews, pumpkin seeds, and sesame seeds contain significant amounts of this essential mineral. Snack on these nutritious options or sprinkle them over salads, yogurt, or other dishes to increase your iron intake.

Leafy Green Vegetables: Dark leafy greens like spinach, kale, Swiss chard, and collard greens are not only rich in iron but also packed with other essential nutrients. Incorporate these greens into salads, stir-fries, smoothies, or soups to boost your iron levels.

Fortified Foods: Fortified foods are products that have nutrients added to them. Look for iron-fortified cereals, bread, or plant-based milk alternatives to increase your iron intake. Check the nutrition labels to ensure they contain iron and other important nutrients.

Strategies for Maximizing Iron Absorption

Pair Iron-Rich Foods with Vitamin C: Consuming iron-rich foods alongside vitamin C-rich foods can enhance iron absorption. Include citrus fruits, berries, tomatoes, bell peppers, or foods fortified with vitamin C in your meals. Consider adding a squeeze of lemon juice to iron-rich dishes or enjoying a fruit salad after your meal to optimize iron absorption.

Avoid Consuming Iron with Inhibitors: Some foods and substances can inhibit iron absorption. Try to separate the consumption of iron-rich foods from these inhibitors by a few hours to maximize iron absorption.

- **Phytates**: Found in whole grains, legumes, nuts, and seeds, phytates can bind to iron and hinder its absorption. Soaking, fermenting, or sprouting these foods can help reduce the phytate content and improve iron absorption.

- **Oxalates**: Foods high in oxalates, such as spinach, beet greens, rhubarb, and chocolate, can inhibit iron absorption. Cooking these foods can reduce the oxalate content and improve iron availability.

- **Polyphenols**: Certain polyphenols found in tea, coffee, red wine, and some fruits and vegetables can hinder iron absorption. Consuming these beverages or foods separately from iron-rich meals can minimize the inhibitory effect.

- **Calcium**: Calcium can interfere with iron absorption when consumed together. Dairy products, calcium-fortified foods, and calcium supplements should be consumed separately from iron-rich foods to enhance iron absorption.

- **Tannins**: Tannins are naturally occurring compounds found in tea, coffee, red wine, and some fruits, such as grapes and pomegranates. They can inhibit iron absorption. Drinking tea or coffee between meals, rather than with iron-rich foods, can help minimize the impact.

- **High-Fiber Foods**: Foods rich in insoluble fiber, such as bran and whole grains, can reduce iron absorption. However, consuming them as part of a balanced diet is still important for overall health. Combining these foods with sources of vitamin C can enhance iron absorption.

Cooking in Cast Iron Cookware: Cooking foods in cast iron cookware can increase the iron content of the food. The iron from the cookware leaches into the food during cooking, providing an additional source of dietary iron. However, it is important to note that this method primarily enhances the non-heme iron content, so combining it with vitamin C-rich foods remains beneficial.

Consult with Your Healthcare Team: If you are experiencing iron deficiency or anemia, it is important to consult with your healthcare team, including your doctor and renal dietitian.

They can evaluate your specific iron needs, conduct relevant lab tests, and recommend appropriate iron supplementation if necessary.

BALANCING IRON INTAKE WITH OTHER DIETARY CONSIDERATIONS

While increasing iron intake is important, it's crucial to balance it with other dietary considerations. Here are a few points to consider:

Phosphorus and Potassium: Some high-iron foods, especially animal-based sources, may also be high in phosphorus or potassium. If you have restrictions on these minerals due to your kidney health, choose iron-rich foods that align with your dietary needs. Consult with your healthcare team or renal dietitian for personalized guidance on incorporating iron-rich options into your meal plan while managing your phosphorus and potassium levels.

Fluid Intake: Adequate hydration is important for overall kidney health, but it can also affect iron absorption. Ensure you maintain appropriate fluid intake as advised by your healthcare team to support optimal iron absorption.

Individual Needs: Each person's iron needs may vary based on factors such as kidney function, anemia severity, and underlying health conditions. Work closely with your healthcare team to determine your specific iron requirements and dietary recommendations tailored to your unique needs.

IRON SUPPLEMENTS

In some cases, iron supplements may be necessary for individuals with iron deficiency anemia or those who cannot meet their iron needs through diet alone.

Consultation with Healthcare Provider: Before considering iron supplements, it is essential to consult with your healthcare provider. They will evaluate your iron levels through blood tests and determine if supplementation is necessary. Self-supplementation without medical guidance can lead to iron overload, which can be harmful.

Types of Iron Supplements: There are different types of iron supplements available, including ferrous sulfate, ferrous gluconate, and ferrous fumarate. Your healthcare provider will recommend the most appropriate form based on your specific needs and tolerability.

Pros and Cons of Iron Supplements: Iron supplements can effectively raise iron levels and improve symptoms of anemia. However, they may cause side effects such as constipation, nausea, or stomach upset. Your healthcare provider will discuss the benefits and potential risks of iron supplementation with you as well as help you find the one best for you.

Importance of Monitoring: If you are prescribed iron supplements, it is crucial to have regular follow-up appointments with your healthcare provider to monitor your iron levels. This ensures that the supplementation is effective and safe.

Remember, iron supplements should only be taken under the guidance of a healthcare professional and as recommended. **It is not advisable to self-prescribe** or exceed the recommended dosage, as excessive iron intake can be harmful.

By incorporating iron-rich foods into your kidney-friendly diet, optimizing iron absorption, and considering iron supplementation when necessary and guided by your healthcare team, you can support your iron levels and manage anemia effectively.

SUPPLEMENTS: A PRACTICAL APPROACH

In this chapter, we will explore the use of supplements in kidney disease management. We will discuss the importance of prioritizing real food sources over supplements, the potential benefits of renal multivitamins, and specifically, the features of ProRenal+D, a renal multivitamin that you take as recommended by your doctor and renal dietitian. Let's delve into the practical considerations surrounding supplements in the context of kidney health.

EXPLORING THE USE OF SUPPLEMENTS IN KIDNEY DISEASE MANAGEMENT

Supplements have gained popularity as people seek to optimize their nutrition and address specific health concerns, including kidney disease. However, it is essential to approach supplement use in kidney disease management with caution and understanding. Let's delve deeper into the considerations and factors to keep in mind when exploring the use of supplements.

Nutrient Deficiencies and Individual Needs:

In kidney disease, certain nutrients may become deficient

due to decreased intake, impaired absorption, or increased losses. Common nutrient deficiencies in kidney disease include vitamin D, B vitamins (especially B12 and folate), iron, calcium, and zinc. In such cases, supplements may be necessary to help address these deficiencies.

However, it is crucial to note that not all individuals with kidney disease will have the same nutrient deficiencies. The extent and type of nutrient deficiencies can vary depending on factors such as the stage of kidney disease, individual health status, dietary habits, and other underlying conditions. Therefore, it is essential to work with your healthcare team to identify and address your specific nutrient needs through targeted supplementation when necessary.

Individualized Approach:

Supplement use in kidney disease management should be individualized based on a comprehensive assessment by healthcare professionals, such as doctors and renal dietitians. They will consider factors such as your lab results, medical history, dietary intake, and overall health status to determine if supplements are needed and recommend appropriate dosages.

It is important to emphasize that indiscriminate and excessive supplement use can be detrimental to health. Mega-dosing of vitamins and minerals, without medical supervision, can lead to imbalances, toxicity, and potential harm. Therefore, it is crucial to consult with your healthcare team before starting any supplements and to follow their recommendations closely.

Quality and Safety:

When considering supplements, it is vital to select

reputable brands that adhere to good manufacturing practices and undergo third-party testing. This ensures that the supplements are of high quality, free from contaminants, and accurately labeled. Your healthcare team can provide guidance on trusted supplement brands and help you make informed choices.

Real Food Sources as the Foundation:

While supplements may play a role in addressing specific nutrient deficiencies, it is important to prioritize obtaining nutrients from real food sources whenever possible. Whole foods offer a complex matrix of nutrients, fiber, and bioactive compounds that work synergistically to support health. They also provide additional benefits such as phytochemicals, antioxidants, and dietary fiber, which are not found in isolated supplements.

A well-balanced diet consisting of a variety of nutrient-dense whole foods, including fruits, vegetables, whole grains, lean proteins, and healthy fats, should form the foundation of your nutrition. This approach ensures a comprehensive nutrient intake and supports overall health while minimizing reliance on supplements.

Remember, supplement use should always be guided by healthcare professionals who can assess your specific nutrient needs, evaluate the benefits and risks, and provide individualized recommendations based on your unique circumstances.

RECOMMENDATIONS FOR REAL FOOD SOURCES OVER SUPPLEMENTS

When it comes to meeting your nutritional needs, obtaining

nutrients from real food sources is generally preferred over relying solely on supplements. Real foods provide a myriad of benefits beyond isolated nutrients, including fiber, antioxidants, phytochemicals, and a balanced combination of essential nutrients. Here, we will explore the reasons why real food sources should be prioritized and offer recommendations for incorporating them into your kidney-friendly diet.

Nutrient Synergy and Bioavailability:

Real food sources offer a natural combination of essential nutrients in a bioavailable form. Nutrients work together synergistically, meaning they interact and enhance each other's absorption and utilization in the body. For example, vitamin C enhances the absorption of iron from plant-based sources, while the presence of healthy fats can aid the absorption of fat-soluble vitamins like vitamin D and vitamin E.

By consuming whole foods, you benefit from the intricate balance of nutrients that nature provides, optimizing nutrient absorption and utilization. This comprehensive nutrient package supports your overall health and well-being, including kidney health.

Fiber and Micronutrients:

Whole foods, such as fruits, vegetables, whole grains, legumes, and nuts, are rich in dietary fiber. Fiber plays a crucial role in digestive health, promoting regular bowel movements, preventing constipation, and supporting the growth of beneficial gut bacteria.

Additionally, real foods are abundant in micronutrients, including vitamins and minerals, which are essential for numerous bodily functions. These micronutrients work together in intricate pathways and play a role in maintaining optimal health.

Antioxidants and Phytochemicals:

Real foods are packed with antioxidants and phytochemicals, which are bioactive compounds that have protective and health-promoting properties. Antioxidants help neutralize harmful free radicals in the body, reducing oxidative stress and inflammation, which are key factors in the progression of chronic diseases, including kidney disease.

Phytochemicals, found in colorful fruits and vegetables, herbs, spices, and other plant-based foods, have been shown to possess various health benefits. They have anti-inflammatory, antimicrobial, and anticancer properties, and they support overall health and immune function.

Dietary Variety and Enjoyment:

Incorporating a diverse range of real foods into your diet provides a broader spectrum of nutrients, flavors, and textures. Variety not only ensures a comprehensive nutrient intake but also adds enjoyment and satisfaction to your meals. Exploring different foods and flavors can make healthy eating more enjoyable and sustainable in the long run.

Tips for Incorporating Real Food Sources:

Choose Whole, Unprocessed Foods: Opt for whole grains, fresh fruits and vegetables, lean proteins, legumes, and nuts. Minimize consumption of processed and packaged foods, as they tend to be high in sodium, phosphorus additives, and unhealthy fats.

Prioritize Plant-Based Foods: Plant-based foods, such as fruits, vegetables, whole grains, legumes, and nuts, are naturally low in sodium, phosphorus, and saturated fats, making them excellent choices for kidney health. Aim to include a variety of plant-based foods in your meals.

Cook at Home: Preparing meals at home gives you more control over the ingredients you use. Experiment with different recipes and cooking methods to enhance the flavors of whole foods without relying on excessive salt, sugar, or unhealthy fats.

Embrace Seasonal and Local Produce: Choose seasonal and locally sourced fruits and vegetables whenever possible. They are often fresher, tastier, and packed with nutrients.

Collaborate with a Renal Dietitian: Work closely with a renal dietitian who can provide personalized guidance and meal planning strategies to ensure you meet your nutritional needs through real food sources.

Remember, while supplements may play a role in addressing specific nutrient deficiencies, they should not replace the rich array of nutrients and health benefits that real food sources provide. By prioritizing real food choices and incorporating a wide variety of nutrient-dense options, you can optimize your kidney health and overall well-being.

BENEFITS OF RENAL MULTIVITAMINS AND WHEN THEY MAY BE BENEFICIAL

A renal multivitamin offers several benefits specifically tailored to the nutritional needs of individuals with kidney disease. Unlike traditional multivitamins, which may not take into account the unique considerations of kidney health, renal multivitamins are formulated to support the overall well-being of individuals with compromised kidney function. Here are some key reasons why a renal multivitamin is preferred over a traditional multivitamin for people with kidney disease:

Kidney-Friendly Nutrient Balance: A renal multivitamin is designed to provide appropriate amounts of essential vitamins and minerals while considering the restrictions and requirements of kidney disease. It takes into account the delicate balance of nutrients necessary to support kidney health and optimize overall well-being.

Reduced Levels of Certain Nutrients: Kidney disease can alter the way the body handles and eliminates certain nutrients. For example, individuals with kidney disease may need to limit their intake of phosphorus, potassium, or sodium. Renal multivitamins are formulated with reduced levels of these nutrients to help maintain their balance within the body and prevent potential complications associated with excessive intake.

Adjusted Vitamin D Levels: Vitamin D plays a critical role in bone health, immune function, and overall well-being. However, impaired kidney function can disrupt the activation of vitamin D. Renal multivitamins often contain adjusted levels of vitamin D to help address deficiencies commonly seen in individuals with kidney disease.

Consideration of Medications and Medical Conditions: People with kidney disease often have other underlying medical conditions and may be taking multiple medications. A renal multivitamin takes into account these factors, considering potential interactions and ensuring the formulation is safe and appropriate for individuals with kidney disease and their specific medical profiles.

Personalized Nutritional Support: Renal multivitamins are often recommended by healthcare professionals who have a deep understanding of kidney health and the nutritional needs of individuals with kidney disease. They can provide personalized guidance based on individual lab results, medical history, and specific nutritional requirements, ensuring that the renal multivitamin aligns with each person's unique needs.

It is important to note that traditional multivitamins are generally not recommended for individuals with kidney disease because they may contain higher levels of certain minerals (such as phosphorus or potassium) that could potentially be harmful to kidney function or disrupt the delicate nutrient balance required by individuals with compromised kidneys.

PRORENAL+D: A RENAL MULTIVITAMIN FOR KIDNEY HEALTH

ProRenal+D is a specific brand of renal multivitamin supplement formulated for individuals with kidney disease. It is designed to provide essential vitamins and minerals while taking into consideration the unique nutritional needs of individuals with compromised kidney function. This is the renal multivitamin that I personally take as recommended by my doctor and renal dietitian. You can learn more about ProRenal+D at the http://www.myprorenal.com/ website.

ProRenal+D is specially formulated to support kidney health and address common nutrient deficiencies often associated with kidney disease. It typically contains a combination of vitamins and minerals, including B vitamins, vitamin C, vitamin D, vitamin E, iron, zinc, and others. These nutrients are carefully selected to meet the specific requirements of individuals with kidney disease and help maintain optimal health.

One key component of ProRenal+D is vitamin D, which plays a crucial role in bone health and immune function. Individuals with kidney disease often have reduced kidney function, leading to impaired vitamin D synthesis. Supplementing with vitamin D in a controlled manner can help maintain adequate levels and support overall well-being.

It is important to note that ProRenal+D, like any other supplement, should be used under the guidance and supervision of your healthcare team, including your doctor and renal dietitian. They will evaluate your specific nutrient needs, consider your medical history and lab results, and determine if a renal multivitamin supplement like ProRenal+D is appropriate for you.

Remember, it is crucial to involve your healthcare team in decisions regarding supplement use, including renal multivitamins. They have the expertise to evaluate your unique nutritional needs, assess any potential interactions with medications, and ensure that supplement use aligns with your overall kidney health management plan.

While renal multivitamins may provide specific benefits for individuals with kidney disease, it is important to note that they should not replace a well-balanced diet. Real food sources remain the foundation for meeting nutritional needs whenever possible.

WHAT ABOUT HERBAL AND OTHER SUPPLEMENTS

It is crucial for individuals with kidney disease to be cautious when considering herbal and other supplements. While some supplements may claim to have miraculous effects on kidney health, it is important to recognize that these claims are often unsubstantiated and can be misleading. Taking supplements without proper guidance from your healthcare team or dietitian can pose significant risks and potentially accelerate the decline of kidney function. This section aims to shed light on the dangers and concerns associated with unregulated supplements.

False Claims and Unproven Health Claims: Many supplements on the market make bold assertions about curing kidney disease, restoring kidney function, or improving overall kidney health. However, it is essential to approach such claims with skepticism and rely on evidence-based information. The truth is, there is no magic pill or supplement that can reverse kidney damage or cure kidney disease.

Lack of Regulation and Quality Control: Unlike prescription medications, supplements are not subject to the same rigorous testing and regulation by regulatory authorities. This means that the safety, efficacy, and quality of supplements can vary greatly. Without proper regulation, it is challenging to ensure the purity, potency, and accuracy of the ingredients listed on supplement labels.

Potential Interactions and Side Effects: Supplements can interact with medications or other treatments, potentially leading to adverse effects or interfering with their efficacy. Moreover, certain supplements may contain substances that can be harmful to the kidneys or exacerbate existing kidney problems. It is crucial to discuss any supplement use with your healthcare team to assess potential risks and benefits.

Accelerated Kidney Function Decline: In some cases, taking unproven supplements can actually harm kidney function. Certain substances in supplements may place additional stress on the kidneys or interfere with their normal functioning. This can lead to an acceleration of kidney function decline and potentially worsen overall health outcomes.

Importance of Medical Guidance: The safest approach for individuals with kidney disease is to consult with their healthcare team or a registered dietitian before considering any supplements. These professionals can provide personalized advice based on your specific health condition, medications, and individual needs. They can guide you on appropriate nutritional strategies and help you make informed decisions regarding supplement use, if necessary.

It is vital to prioritize evidence-based medical care and rely on the expertise of your healthcare team when it comes to managing your kidney health. Taking unregulated supplements based on false claims can be not only ineffective but also potentially harmful. Trusting your healthcare team and following their recommendations is key to promoting kidney health and overall well-being.

FAT-SOLUBLE AND WATER-SOLUBLE VITAMINS: ESSENTIAL NUTRIENTS FOR KIDNEY HEALTH

In this chapter, we will explore the importance of fat-soluble and water-soluble vitamins in supporting kidney health. Understanding these vitamins, their food sources, and how to balance vitamin intake with kidney-friendly guidelines is crucial for maintaining optimal nutrition and overall well-being.

UNDERSTANDING THE IMPORTANCE OF FAT-SOLUBLE AND WATER-SOLUBLE VITAMINS

Fat-soluble vitamins and water-soluble vitamins are both essential for maintaining good health, but they differ in their properties and functions within the body. Let's delve deeper into the importance of each type of vitamin:

Fat-Soluble Vitamins:

Vitamin A: Vitamin A is crucial for vision, immune function, and cellular growth and differentiation. It plays a key role in maintaining the health of epithelial tissues, which include the skin and the lining of the respiratory, digestive, and urinary tracts. Vitamin A also supports the normal functioning of the retina, contributing to optimal eyesight.

Vitamin D: Vitamin D is essential for calcium absorption and utilization, playing a vital role in bone health. It helps regulate calcium and phosphorus levels in the body, promoting their absorption from the digestive tract and maintaining proper mineralization of bones and teeth. Additionally, vitamin D is involved in immune function and cell growth regulation.

Vitamin E: Vitamin E acts as a potent antioxidant, protecting cells from oxidative damage caused by free radicals. It helps maintain the integrity of cell membranes and supports immune function. Vitamin E also plays a role in the formation of red blood cells and the dilation of blood vessels, contributing to cardiovascular health.

Vitamin K: Vitamin K is primarily involved in blood clotting and bone metabolism. It plays a critical role in the synthesis of proteins that facilitate proper blood coagulation, preventing excessive bleeding. Additionally, vitamin K is essential for bone mineralization, helping to maintain strong and healthy bones.

Water-Soluble Vitamins:

Vitamin C: Vitamin C is known for its antioxidant properties and its role in collagen synthesis, a protein that supports the structure of tissues, skin, and blood vessels. Vitamin C also aids in iron absorption, supports immune function, and contributes to wound healing. It acts as a powerful antioxidant, protecting cells from damage caused by free radicals.

B-Complex Vitamins: The B-complex vitamins, including thiamin (B1), riboflavin (B2), niacin (B3), vitamin B6, folate (B9), and vitamin B12, play crucial roles in energy metabolism, nervous system function, and red blood cell production. These vitamins are involved in converting food into energy, maintaining healthy skin and hair, promoting brain health, and supporting DNA synthesis.

It's important to note that fat-soluble vitamins are stored in the body's fatty tissues, whereas water-soluble vitamins are not stored and are excreted through urine. Therefore, fat-soluble vitamins have the potential to accumulate to toxic levels if consumed in excess, while water-soluble vitamins require regular intake to meet the body's needs.

A well-balanced diet that includes a variety of foods can help ensure adequate intake of both fat-soluble and water-soluble vitamins. However, it is important to work with your healthcare team, including a renal dietitian, to tailor your vitamin intake based on your specific kidney health needs and overall health status. They can provide guidance on suitable food sources, portion sizes, and potential supplementation if necessary.

FOOD SOURCES AND CONSIDERATIONS FOR OPTIMAL VITAMIN INTAKE

Obtaining vitamins from natural food sources is generally the best way to ensure optimal nutrient intake and support kidney health. Let's explore the food sources and considerations for obtaining vitamins from your diet:

Fat-Soluble Vitamins:

Vitamin A:

Food Sources: Rich sources of vitamin A include liver, fish oil, dairy products, fortified plant-based milk, carrots, sweet potatoes, spinach, kale, and other dark leafy greens. These foods contain beta-carotene, which the body converts into vitamin A.

Considerations: It is important to maintain an appropriate intake level of vitamin A, as excessive consumption can lead to toxicity. Consult with your healthcare team, including a renal dietitian, to determine the right amount of vitamin A based on your specific needs.

Vitamin D:

Food Sources: Natural sources of vitamin D include fatty fish like salmon and mackerel, cod liver oil, egg yolks, and fortified foods such as milk, cereal, or plant-based milk alternatives. Sun exposure also helps the body synthesize vitamin D.

Considerations: Individuals with kidney disease often require careful monitoring of vitamin D levels, as impaired kidney function can affect vitamin D metabolism. Your healthcare team may recommend regular monitoring and potentially vitamin D supplementation to maintain adequate levels.

Vitamin E:

Food Sources: Good sources of vitamin E include nuts (almonds, hazelnuts, peanuts), seeds (sunflower seeds, pumpkin seeds), vegetable oils (sunflower oil, safflower oil, wheat germ oil), spinach, and fortified cereals.

Considerations: Selecting unsaturated fats and oils as sources of vitamin E is important to maintain a healthy balance of fats in the diet. It's advisable to moderate intake if you have specific dietary restrictions or conditions that require limited fat intake.

Vitamin K:

Food Sources: Dark leafy greens such as kale, spinach, broccoli, Brussels sprouts, and cabbage are excellent sources of vitamin K. Liver and fermented foods like sauerkraut also contain vitamin K.

Considerations: Individuals taking blood-thinning medications (anticoagulants) need to maintain consistent vitamin K intake. Consult with your healthcare team to determine the appropriate level of vitamin K intake based on your specific medication regimen.

Water-Soluble Vitamins:

Vitamin C:

Food Sources: Citrus fruits (oranges, lemons, grapefruits), strawberries, kiwi, bell peppers, broccoli, tomatoes, and leafy greens are rich sources of vitamin C.

Considerations: Including vitamin C-rich foods in your diet is important as they can enhance iron absorption. Ensure a variety of fruits and vegetables to obtain a wide range of nutrients.

B-Complex Vitamins:

Food Sources: B-complex vitamins can be found in whole grains, legumes, leafy greens, meat, poultry, fish, eggs, dairy products, and fortified foods. Consuming a varied and balanced diet can help meet the requirements for these vitamins.

Considerations: If you have dietary restrictions or specific nutrient needs, such as limiting phosphorus or potassium, work with your renal dietitian to choose suitable food sources that meet your individual requirements.

When considering optimal vitamin intake, it is important to focus on consuming a well-balanced diet that incorporates a variety of nutrient-dense foods. This approach helps ensure you receive a broad spectrum of vitamins and minerals. However, the nutritional needs of individuals with kidney disease can vary, so consulting with your healthcare team, including a renal dietitian, is crucial. They can help you personalize your diet, taking into account your kidney health, underlying conditions, and specific nutrient requirements, to optimize your vitamin intake and support your overall well-being.

BALANCING VITAMIN NEEDS WITH KIDNEY-FRIENDLY GUIDELINES

When managing kidney disease, it is important to strike a balance between meeting your vitamin needs and adhering to kidney-friendly guidelines. Here are some considerations for achieving this balance:

Consult with Your Healthcare Team: Collaborate with your healthcare team, including your doctor and renal dietitian, to determine your specific vitamin needs based on your kidney function, lab results, and overall health status. They can provide personalized guidance and recommend appropriate dietary modifications or supplementation.

Portion Control and Moderation: While vitamins are essential for overall health, excessive intake of certain vitamins can be harmful, especially for individuals with kidney disease. Adhering to portion control and moderation is key. Pay attention to recommended serving sizes and avoid overconsumption of vitamin supplements or fortified foods.

Phosphorus Considerations: Individuals with kidney disease often need to limit their phosphorus intake. Certain sources of vitamins, such as organ meats, dairy products, and whole grains, can be high in phosphorus. Work with your renal dietitian to identify alternative food sources or ways to reduce phosphorus content while still meeting your vitamin requirements.

Potassium Considerations: Some foods rich in vitamins, such as bananas, oranges, tomatoes, and certain leafy greens, may also be high in potassium. Depending on your individual potassium needs, your healthcare team may recommend portion control or alternative food choices to manage your potassium intake.

Sodium Considerations: Foods fortified with vitamins, such as processed snacks or canned goods, may be high in sodium. Excessive sodium intake can negatively affect blood pressure and kidney health. Read food labels carefully and opt for low-sodium or sodium-free alternatives whenever possible.

Supplement Usage: If it is determined that you need vitamin supplementation, consult with your healthcare team for appropriate recommendations. They can guide you on choosing kidney-friendly supplements and ensure that they do not interfere with any medications you may be taking.

Regular Monitoring: Regular monitoring of your vitamin levels through blood tests is important to assess any deficiencies or excesses. This allows your healthcare team to make necessary adjustments to your diet or supplementation regimen.

Individualized Approach: Each person's nutritional needs and vitamin requirements may vary based on factors such as kidney function, underlying health conditions, and medication usage. It is essential to work closely with your healthcare team to develop an individualized approach that

meets your specific needs while considering kidney-friendly
guidelines.

THE ROLE OF HEALTHY FATS: UNDERSTANDING AND INCORPORATING GOOD FATS

In this chapter, we delve into the importance of healthy fats for kidney health and how to incorporate them into your kidney-friendly diet. While fats are often associated with negative connotations, it's crucial to understand that not all fats are created equal. Healthy fats play a vital role in supporting various bodily functions, including kidney health. By identifying sources of healthy fats and learning to balance fat intake with other dietary considerations, you can optimize your overall well-being.

IMPORTANCE OF HEALTHY FATS FOR KIDNEY HEALTH

The importance of healthy fats for kidney health cannot be overstated. While fats have long been associated with negative health effects, it is crucial to understand that not all fats are harmful. In fact, incorporating the right types of fats into your kidney-friendly diet can offer numerous benefits and support optimal kidney function.

Energy and Nutrient Absorption: Healthy fats, specifically monounsaturated and polyunsaturated fats, serve as a concentrated source of energy. They provide essential fatty acids, such as omega-3 and omega-6, which are necessary for various bodily functions. These fats also play a vital role in the absorption of fat-soluble vitamins, including vitamins A, D, E, and K. These vitamins are crucial for maintaining overall health and supporting kidney function.

Heart Health: Kidney disease is often associated with an increased risk of cardiovascular complications. Consuming healthy fats can help mitigate this risk and promote heart health. Monounsaturated fats, found in foods like avocados and olive oil, have been shown to improve lipid profiles by increasing levels of high-density lipoprotein (HDL) cholesterol, often referred to as "good" cholesterol. This can help reduce the risk of heart disease and protect against atherosclerosis.

Inflammation Reduction: Chronic inflammation is a common issue in kidney disease. Incorporating healthy fats can help combat inflammation and promote better overall health. Omega-3 fatty acids, present in fatty fish like salmon and sardines, have potent anti-inflammatory properties. They can help reduce the production of inflammatory markers in the body, leading to improved kidney function and reduced risk of complications.

Hormone Production and Regulation: Healthy fats are essential for the production and regulation of hormones in the body. Hormones play a crucial role in various physiological processes, including kidney function. Consuming adequate amounts of healthy fats supports the proper functioning of hormonal systems, contributing to better overall health and kidney function.

Nutrient Density: Many healthy fats are found in nutrient-dense foods that offer additional health benefits. For example, avocados are not only a source of healthy fats but also provide dietary fiber, vitamins, minerals, and antioxidants. Incorporating these nutrient-rich foods into your diet helps support overall health and provides a wide range of essential nutrients.

It is important to note that while healthy fats offer significant benefits, moderation is key. While they provide essential nutrients and promote overall health, consuming excessive amounts of fats can lead to weight gain and other health issues. Working with a renal dietitian can help determine the appropriate amount of healthy fats to incorporate into your kidney-friendly diet, considering your specific dietary needs, kidney function, and overall health status.

IDENTIFYING SOURCES OF HEALTHY FATS AND THEIR BENEFITS

Identifying sources of healthy fats and understanding their benefits is key to incorporating them into a kidney-friendly diet. Here are some examples of healthy fat sources and their specific benefits:

Avocados: Avocados are rich in monounsaturated fats, which have been shown to improve heart health by reducing levels of harmful LDL cholesterol and increasing levels of beneficial HDL cholesterol. They also contain fiber, which aids in digestion and promotes satiety. Avocados are also a good source of vitamin E, an antioxidant that helps protect cells from damage.

Nuts and Seeds: Almonds, walnuts, flaxseeds, and chia seeds are excellent sources of healthy fats, including omega-3 fatty acids. These fats have anti-inflammatory properties and can help reduce the risk of heart disease. Nuts and seeds also provide fiber, protein, and various vitamins and minerals, making them a nutrient-dense addition to a kidney-friendly diet.

Olive Oil: Extra virgin olive oil is a staple in Mediterranean cuisine and is a rich source of monounsaturated fats. It has been associated with numerous health benefits, including reducing the risk of heart disease, improving insulin sensitivity, and reducing inflammation. Olive oil also contains antioxidants that protect against oxidative stress and inflammation.

Fatty Fish: Fatty fish like salmon, mackerel, and sardines are excellent sources of omega-3 fatty acids. These fats have been shown to lower inflammation, improve heart health, and support brain function. Consuming fatty fish regularly can help reduce the risk of heart disease and promote overall well-being.

Nut Butters: Natural nut butters, such as peanut butter, almond butter, and cashew butter, offer a tasty and convenient way to incorporate healthy fats into your diet. They are a good source of monounsaturated and polyunsaturated fats, as well as protein. Nut butters also provide essential vitamins and minerals like vitamin E, magnesium, and potassium.

Seeds: Sesame seeds, pumpkin seeds, and sunflower seeds

are nutrient-dense sources of healthy fats. They contain a combination of monounsaturated and polyunsaturated fats, as well as fiber, vitamins, and minerals. Seeds are versatile and can be added to salads, yogurt, or smoothies to enhance flavor and nutrient content.

BALANCING FAT INTAKE WITH OTHER DIETARY CONSIDERATIONS

Balancing fat intake with other dietary considerations is crucial for maintaining a kidney-friendly diet that supports overall health. Here are some important factors to consider when it comes to incorporating fats into your diet:

Portion Control: While healthy fats offer numerous benefits, they are calorie-dense. It's essential to practice portion control to avoid consuming excessive calories, which can lead to weight gain and other health issues. Be mindful of serving sizes and aim to incorporate fats in moderation.

Quality Matters: Choose high-quality sources of fats that are minimally processed and free from additives, trans fats, and unhealthy oils. Opt for natural sources of fats like avocados, nuts, seeds, and cold-pressed oils. Avoid foods high in unhealthy fats, such as processed snacks, fried foods, and commercially baked goods.

Consider Overall Diet: Balancing fat intake with other dietary considerations means looking at your diet as a whole. Ensure you have a well-rounded eating plan that includes a variety of nutrient-dense foods from different food groups. Incorporate fruits, vegetables, lean proteins, whole grains, and low-fat dairy products to provide a wide range of essential nutrients.

Individualize Your Diet: Every individual's dietary needs and health conditions may vary. Work with a renal dietitian to personalize your fat intake based on your specific nutritional needs, kidney function, and any other underlying health conditions. They can provide guidance and support in developing a balanced meal plan that aligns with your unique requirements.

Regular Monitoring: Regularly monitor your lipid profile and consult with your healthcare team to assess the impact of your dietary choices on your overall health. Monitoring your blood lipid levels, including cholesterol and triglycerides, can help determine if adjustments in fat intake are necessary. This can be done through routine blood tests and discussions with your healthcare provider.

Emphasize Healthy Sources: Prioritize sources of healthy fats such as avocados, nuts, seeds, olive oil, and fatty fish. These foods not only provide healthy fats but also offer additional nutritional benefits like vitamins, minerals, and antioxidants. Incorporating these foods into your diet helps ensure that you receive the essential nutrients your body needs.

By understanding the role of healthy fats, identifying their sources, and balancing fat intake with other dietary considerations, you can incorporate good fats into your kidney-friendly diet to support optimal kidney health and overall well-being.

THE BEST DIET FOR CKD

The best diet for kidney disease is one that addresses the unique nutritional needs of each individual while also promoting overall health and well-being. A heart-healthy, individualized diet rich in plant-based foods is the key to managing kidney disease and slowing its progression. In this chapter, we will discuss the importance of working with a dietitian to customize a kidney-friendly diet, the benefits of plant-based eating, and the suitability of the DASH diet for many kidney patients.

THE IMPORTANCE OF A HEART-HEALTHY, INDIVIDUALIZED DIET

A well-rounded, heart-healthy diet is of paramount importance in managing kidney disease and preserving overall health. It is vital to understand that one-size-fits-all diets or food lists alone **do not work**. Each person's dietary requirements must be individualized and adjusted based on their health, existing conditions such as diabetes or high blood pressure, their lifestyle, activity level, and lab results. By emphasizing foods that promote cardiovascular health and tailoring the diet to meet each individual's unique needs, it becomes possible to slow the progression of kidney disease and enhance the quality of life.

WORKING WITH A DIETITIAN FOR A CUSTOMIZED KIDNEY-

As a kidney health coach, I cannot stress enough the importance of working closely with a dietitian to develop a personalized meal plan. A dietitian specializes in understanding the complex nutritional requirements of individuals with kidney disease and can provide the education and tools necessary to make confident, healthy eating choices. Some benefits of working with a dietitian include:

Personalized guidance: A dietitian can assess your unique nutritional needs based on factors such as age, weight, lifestyle, and stage of kidney disease. This personalized approach ensures that your diet is tailored to meet your specific requirements.

Ongoing support: As your kidney function changes, so too will your dietary needs. A dietitian can provide ongoing support and adjustments to your meal plan to ensure that it remains effective and appropriate for your changing needs.

Education: A dietitian can teach you about the relationship between nutrition and kidney health, helping you to make informed decisions about the foods you consume.

Confidence: By working with a dietitian, you can feel confident in your ability to make healthy eating choices that support your kidney health and overall well-being.

THE BENEFITS OF PLANT-BASED EATING FOR KIDNEY PATIENTS

A diet rich in plant-based foods offers numerous benefits for individuals with kidney disease. Plant-based foods are naturally low in sodium, potassium, and phosphorus, making them an ideal choice for a kidney-friendly diet. Some additional benefits of plant-based eating include:

Improved cardiovascular health: A plant-based diet can help lower blood pressure, cholesterol levels, and reduce the risk of heart disease, which is especially important for kidney patients.

Better blood sugar control: Plant-based foods are rich in fiber and low in added sugars, which can help stabilize blood sugar levels and manage diabetes, a common risk factor for kidney disease.

Reduced inflammation: A diet rich in plant-based foods can help reduce inflammation in the body, which is associated with kidney disease progression.

Enhanced gut health: Plant-based foods, particularly those high in fiber, can improve gut health and promote a healthy balance of gut bacteria, which can be beneficial for individuals with kidney disease.

THE DASH DIET: A COMMON STARTING POINT FOR KIDNEY PATIENTS

The DASH (Dietary Approaches to Stop Hypertension) diet is a well-studied and highly recommended eating plan that has been shown to promote heart health and effectively manage blood pressure. While initially developed to lower blood pressure, the DASH diet offers several benefits for individuals with chronic kidney disease (CKD) as well. The key aspects of the DASH diet and its benefits for those with CKD:

Emphasis on Fruits and Vegetables: The DASH diet encourages the consumption of fruits and vegetables, which are excellent sources of essential vitamins, minerals, and antioxidants. They provide fiber and are naturally low in sodium, making them beneficial for managing blood pressure and promoting overall kidney health.

Rich in Whole Grains: The DASH diet includes whole grains such as brown rice, whole wheat bread, and oatmeal. These grains are high in fiber, which aids in digestion and helps control blood sugar levels. Whole grains are also lower in sodium compared to refined grains, making them a kidney-friendly choice.

Moderate Protein Intake: The DASH diet emphasizes lean protein sources like poultry, fish, and legumes. While the DASH diet doesn't specifically limit protein intake, it encourages moderation. This approach can be beneficial for individuals with CKD, as excessive protein intake can put strain on the kidneys.

Low in Sodium: The DASH diet restricts sodium intake, which is crucial for managing blood pressure and fluid balance in individuals with CKD. By reducing sodium intake, the DASH diet can help control hypertension and reduce the risk of fluid retention.

Limited Added Sugars and Sweets: The DASH diet advises limiting the consumption of foods and beverages high in added sugars. This is important for individuals with CKD, as high sugar intake can contribute to diabetes and weight gain, which can negatively impact kidney health.

Encourages Healthy Fats: The DASH diet promotes the consumption of healthy fats, such as those found in nuts, seeds, avocados, and olive oil. These fats are beneficial for heart health and can provide a good source of energy.

The benefits of the DASH diet for those with CKD include:

Balanced and Nutrient-Rich: The DASH diet emphasizes a well-balanced and nutrient-rich eating pattern. It encourages the consumption of a variety of fruits, vegetables, whole grains, lean proteins, and low-fat dairy products. These foods are packed with essential vitamins, minerals, fiber, and antioxidants, which are crucial for overall health and well-being.

Sodium Restriction: A distinctive feature of the DASH diet is its emphasis on limiting sodium intake. High sodium levels can contribute to fluid retention and increase blood pressure. By reducing sodium intake, the DASH diet helps manage blood pressure and prevent fluid buildup in individuals with CKD, who are often advised to limit their sodium intake.

Rich in Potassium, Magnesium, and Calcium: The DASH diet encourages the consumption of foods rich in potassium, magnesium, and calcium, which are vital minerals for maintaining kidney health. Potassium-rich foods like bananas, oranges, spinach, and sweet potatoes can help counteract the negative effects of sodium on blood pressure. Magnesium and calcium are also important for proper muscle function, bone health, and blood pressure regulation.

High Fiber Content: The DASH diet promotes the intake of fiber-rich foods such as whole grains, fruits, vegetables, and legumes. Adequate fiber intake supports digestive health, helps regulate blood sugar levels, and contributes to weight management. Additionally, high-fiber foods can help lower cholesterol levels, reducing the risk of cardiovascular complications in individuals with CKD.

Lean Proteins and Healthy Fats: The DASH diet emphasizes lean protein sources like skinless poultry, fish, legumes, and nuts. These protein sources are lower in saturated fat compared to red meats, which can help manage cholesterol levels and reduce the risk of heart disease. Healthy fats, such as those found in avocados, olive oil, and nuts, are also an essential component of the DASH diet and provide beneficial monounsaturated and polyunsaturated fats.

Portion Control and Mindful Eating: The DASH diet promotes portion control and mindful eating practices. It encourages individuals to be aware of their portion sizes, listen to their body's hunger and fullness cues, and avoid overeating. This approach can help manage weight, prevent overconsumption of calories, and promote overall health.

Flexibility and Adaptability: The DASH diet offers flexibility in food choices, allowing individuals to tailor the plan to their cultural preferences, dietary restrictions, and individual needs. It can be adapted to accommodate different calorie requirements, protein restrictions, and personal taste preferences while still adhering to the core principles of the diet.

While the DASH diet is a popular choice for kidney patients, there are other dietary approaches that can also help manage kidney disease and its complications. Below, we explore some of these diets and the research supporting their use in kidney patients.

1. Mediterranean Diet

The Mediterranean diet is rich in fruits, vegetables, whole grains, legumes, nuts, and olive oil, with moderate amounts of fish, poultry, and dairy products. It emphasizes the consumption of healthy fats, such as monounsaturated and polyunsaturated fats, while limiting the intake of saturated fats and trans fats. The Mediterranean diet is known for its numerous health benefits, including improved cardiovascular health, reduced risk of chronic diseases, and weight management.

A study published in the Clinical Journal of the American Society of Nephrology found that adherence to a Mediterranean-style diet was associated with a lower risk of developing chronic kidney disease (CKD) and a slower decline in kidney function among those with existing CKD (Gutiérrez et al., 2013).

2. Plant-Based Diet

A plant-based diet focuses on consuming whole, minimally processed plant foods, such as fruits, vegetables, whole grains, legumes, nuts, and seeds. This diet is typically low in sodium, saturated fat, and cholesterol, and rich in fiber, antioxidants, and essential nutrients. A plant-based diet can be tailored to include varying amounts of animal products, depending on individual preferences and needs.

A study in the Journal of Renal Nutrition found that CKD patients who followed a plant-based diet experienced improvements in blood pressure, cholesterol, and kidney function, as well as a reduced risk of cardiovascular events and mortality (Chauveau et al., 2013).

3. Low-Protein Diet

A low-protein diet involves restricting the intake of dietary protein to help minimize the workload on the kidneys and reduce the production of waste products. This diet may be recommended for patients with advanced kidney disease or those at risk of rapid progression. Beware, a low-protein diet **can be dangerous** for some kidney patients. It's essential to work closely with a dietitian to ensure that adequate nutrition is maintained while on a low-protein diet.

A systematic review and meta-analysis published in the American Journal of Kidney Diseases found that low-protein diets can help slow the progression of CKD, particularly in patients with diabetes or at high risk of kidney failure (Menon et al., 2009).

4. Ketogenic Diet (KETO)

The ketogenic diet, commonly known as the Keto diet, is a high-fat, low-carbohydrate eating plan that aims to shift the body into a state of ketosis, where it primarily relies on fats for energy instead of carbohydrates. While the Keto diet has gained popularity for its benefits in weight loss and certain medical conditions, it is important to consider its suitability for those with kidney disease.

For those with kidney disease, there are several concerns regarding the Keto diet. The high intake of protein, often a hallmark of the Keto diet, may potentially strain the kidneys, as they play a crucial role in metabolizing and excreting protein waste products. Additionally, the diet's emphasis on fats can lead to an increased intake of saturated and trans fats, which may negatively impact heart health, a common concern for individuals with kidney disease.

Many renal dietitians have experience with the Keto diet and can provide guidance in selecting healthy protein and fat sources. The Kidney Nutrition Institute (KidneyNutritionInstitute.org) and Plant-Powered Kidneys (PlantPoweredKidneys.com) both offer support for those with kidney disease looking to switch to a Keto diet.

The best diet for kidney disease is a heart-healthy, **individualized plan** that prioritizes plant-based foods and takes into account each individual's unique needs. Working with a dietitian to create a customized meal plan is crucial for managing kidney disease and slowing its progression. The DASH diet is a popular, evidence-based option that can be adapted for kidney patients, providing a well-balanced, flexible approach to eating that promotes overall health and well-being.

As a kidney health coach, I strongly encourage kidney patients to seek the guidance of a dietitian. With their expertise and support, you can develop the skills and knowledge necessary to make confident, healthy eating choices that will benefit your kidney health.

KIDNEY DIET FOOD SHOPPING LIST

Navigating the grocery store aisles can be overwhelming, especially when you're following a kidney diet. In this chapter, I'll provide you with a helpful Kidney Diet Food Shopping List, designed to assist those new to the kidney diet in making healthier choices. It's important to note that while this list serves as a starting point, every individual's dietary needs may vary. Working closely with a registered dietitian is essential to personalize your diet and ensure it aligns with your specific health condition, medications, and nutritional requirements.

When it comes to the kidney diet, it's essential to shift our focus from individual items to the **total nutrients we consume**. The goal is to achieve a well-balanced diet that supports kidney health, manages specific nutrient levels, and promotes overall well-being. This shopping list serves as a foundation, offering a variety of nutrient-rich options that can be incorporated into delicious and kidney-friendly meals.

Remember, the kidney diet is **not** about restricting yourself to a long list of forbidden foods. It's about understanding your nutritional needs, making informed choices, and creating a well-rounded eating plan that supports your kidney health. Working with a dietitian will help you understand portion sizes, nutrient balance, and how to adapt the kidney diet to your personal preferences and lifestyle.

So, let this Kidney Diet Food Shopping List be your starting block as you embark on your journey to a healthier lifestyle.

Use it to discover foods that nourish your body, support kidney function, and bring enjoyment to your meals. Embrace the opportunity to work with a dietitian to tailor your diet and make it a sustainable and fulfilling part of your life. Remember, you have the power to take control of your kidney health and thrive on this journey toward well-being.

It is recommended to select brands that do not contain artificial ingredients, preservatives, or GMOs. To control blood sugar, limit carbohydrate portions of starches, fruits, and sweets (those marked with a *). Items marked with a ^ may help prevent or treat Anemia.

Breads/Grains/Cereals*	**Vegetables (½ cup, 1 cup leafy)**
Whole grain versions may be okay to eat. Talk to your dietitian about whether whole grains are okay for you. Look for items with less than 200mg sodium per serving.	Alfalfa or Bean Sprouts
	Arugula
	Asparagus (6 spears) ^
	Bamboo Shoots
	Beets (Canned)
	Bell Peppers
Bagels (Plain, Blueberry, Egg)	Broccoli (Limit)^
	Cabbage (Green and Red)
Bread (White^, Italian, French, Rye^, Sourdough)	Carrots
	Cauliflower
Breadsticks (Plain)	Celery
Bulger	Chayote
Cereals Dry (No Nuts, Dried Fruits, Bran or Granola) ^	Chili Peppers
	Coleslaw *
Cereals Hot (Grits, Oatmeal, Cream of Wheat/Rice) ^	Corn (Limit)
	Cucumber
Cornmeal ^	Dandelion Greens^
Couscous	Eggplant
	Endive
Crackers (Unsalted, Graham, Animal, Oyster)	Green Beans
	Hominy
Croissant	Jalapenos

Crumpets
Dinner Rolls (White^,
Italian, French, light Rye^,
Sourdough)
English Muffins
Grits
Hamburger Buns^
Hotdog Buns^
Kaiser roll
Malt O Meal (Original)
Melba Toast®
Muffins (no nuts, no bran,
no whole wheat)
Naan
Pasta (Noodles, Macaroni,
Spaghetti)^
Pita Bread
Popcorn (Unsalted)
Pretzels (Unsalted)
Quinoa
Rice (White, unseasoned)^
Rice Cakes (low sodium –
read label)
Rice Noodles
Ritz® Crackers (Low
Sodium)
Taco Shells (Corn or Flour)
Tortilla Chips (Unsalted)
Tortillas (Corn or Flour)

Jicama
Kale (Limit)^
Leeks
Lettuce
Mushrooms (Shiitake)
Okra
Onions
Pease (Green or Snow)^
Peppers (Green, Red^,
Yellow)
Radishes
Shallots
Spaghetti Squash
Summer Squash
(Crookneck, Spaghetti)
Tomatillos
Turnips
Water Chestnuts
Watercress
Wax Beans
Zucchini

Fruits* (1 small fruit or ½ cup)	**Seasonings**
Apples	Allspice
Applesauce	Anise
Apricots (Canned)^	Basil
Blackberries	Bay Leaves
	Black Pepper

Blueberries
Boysenberries
Cherries (10)
Crabapples
Cranberries
Fruit Cocktail
Gooseberries
Grapefruit (*Check for medication interaction*)
Grapes
Kumquat
Lemon
Lime
Loganberries
Lychees
Mandarin Oranges
Pears
Peaches^
Pineapple
Pomegranate
Plums
Raspberries
Rhubarb
Strawberries^
Tangerine
Watermelon^

Meat / Protein (3oz) ^
Beef (Lean Cuts)
Beyond Meat ™ Products (watch sodium)
Chicken
Duck
Egg (Whites recommended, real or substitute)
Fish (Wild Salmon, Sea

Caraway Seeds
Cardamom
Celery Seeds
Chili Powder
Chives
Cilantro
Cinnamon
Cloves
Coriander
Crushed Red Pepper Flakes
Cumin
Curry Powder
Dash®
Dill
Extracts (Vanilla, Almond, Peppermint)
Fennel
Fenugreek
Garlic (Fresh or Powder)
Ginger (natural diuretic)
Honey
Horseradish (Root or Powder)
Lemon or Lime Juice
Liquid Smoke®
Mace
Marjoram
Mint
Mustard, Dried
Nutmeg
Onion (Fresh, Powder, Flakes)
Oregano
Paprika
Parsley (natural diuretic)

Bass)	Pimento
Goat	Poppy Seeds
Lamb	Poultry Seasoning
Meat Substitutes – watch for high sodium	Rosemary
Pork (Fresh, Chops or Roast)	Saffron
Shellfish	Sage
Tofu (Soft)	Savory
Tuna (Low Sodium)	Sesame Seeds
Turkey	Tabasco®
Veal	Tarragon
Wild Game	Thyme
	Turmeric
	Vinegar (White, Red Wine, Balsamic, Apple Cider)

<u>**Sweets**</u>***(1 Serving, 1/8 pie, 1 cup)***
Apple Butter
Cake (Sponge, Angel, Pound, Spice, White, Strawberry, Yellow, Lemon, French Vanilla, Vanilla)
Candy Corn
Chewing Gum
Cinnamon Drops / Cinnamon Hearts / Cinnamon Imperials
Cookies (Sugar, Shortbread, Gingersnap, Lemon Cream)
Cotton Candy
Doughnuts (Without Nuts or Chocolate)
Fruit Ice/Frozen Fruit Bars
Gelatin (Not Jell-O® Brand)
Graham Crackers
Gumdrops (5 pieces)
Gummy Bears
Hard Candy (5 pieces)
Honey
Hot Tamales®
Jam/Jelly (Strawberry, Pomegranate, Concord Grape, Blueberry, Mixed Berry)
Jellybeans (9 pieces)
Jolly Rancher®
Jujubes

<u>**Beverages**</u>
Water, Coffee, and Tea are best. The sodas and juices listed are not harmful, but also not beneficial to Kidney Disease patients. Always check the label for Phosphorus or other ingredients!

Apple Cider *
Coffee (Brewed)
Club Soda (limit)
Fruit Punch * / Kool-Aid® / Hi-C® *
Horchata *
Juice (Apple, Cranberry, Grape) *
Lemonade *
Limeade *
Mineral Water
Nectars * (Apricot, Peach, Pear)
Pineapple Juice *
Soda (Cream, Ginger Ale, Grape, Lemon-Lime, Mountain Dew®, Orange, Root Beer) *
Sunny Delight® Citrus Punch *

Tea (Brewed)
True Lime® / True Lemon®

<u>**Dairy**</u> **(1/2 cup)**
Cheese (Swiss^, Brie, Feta, Goat) (1 oz)
Cottage Cheese *

Lifesavers®
Lollipops
Maple Syrup
Marmalade
Marshmallows (5 Large)
Mentos®
Mini Ice Cream Sandwich (Vanilla or Neapolitan)
Newtons (Strawberry, Apple, Blueberry)
Non-Dairy Frozen Dessert (Vanilla, Cookies n Cream, Strawberry)
Peppermints / Mints (not chocolate)
Pie (Apple, Cherry, Lemon, Peach, Blueberry, Lemon Meringue, Rhubarb)
Popsicles (Fruit-Flavored)
Red Licorice / Twizzlers®
Rice Krispies® Treats
Sherbet/Sorbet/Italian Ice (Lemon, Lime, Strawberry, Raspberry, Rainbow)
Skittles®
Sour Patch Kids ™
Starburst®
Strawberry Shortcake
Strudel (Fruit-filled)
Sweet Rolls
Sweet Tarts®
Taffy (not saltwater)
Vanilla Cupcakes

Milk (Skim, 1%, 2%, or whole) (limit) *
Yogurt (limit) *^
Ice Cream (3/4 cup) (limit) *

Dairy Substitutes (Max 1-2 servings per day)

Milk (Rice^, Almond^, Soy^, Unfortified) *
Nondairy Frozen Dessert (Mocha Mix)
Nondairy Creamer (w/o Phosphates) *
Nondairy Dessert Topping (Cool Whip®)

Fats & Extras (Use Sparingly)

Butter or Margarine (Unsalted)
Cream Cheese (Regular or Lite)
Mayonnaise
MCT Oil
Miracle Whip®*
Sour Cream
Vegetable Oils (Canola, Grapeseed or Olive)

Nuts and Seeds

Chia Seeds (1 Tbsp)
Flaxseeds (1 Tbsp)
Macadamia nuts (8 nuts)
Pecans (12 nuts)
Sesame seeds (1 Tbsp)

Vanilla Wafers Werther's® hard candy	

<u>Salad Dressing</u> (2 teaspoons) *Always check sodium levels for <60mg per serving and check for carbs* Unlisted Brand Oil & Vinegar Vinaigrette 3 Zeros Greek Dressing Italian Dressing Mango Dressing Annie's Balsamic Vinaigrette Lite Raspberry Vinaigrette Lite Honey Mustard Vinaigrette (1 tbsp only) Bolthouse Farms Balsamic Honey Mustard Raspberry Merlot Bragg Healthy Vinaigrette Organic Vinaigrette Pomegranate Vinaigrette Compliments ® Sweet Onion Great Value Organic Agave Lemon Flavor Cayenne	**<u>Sauces and Condiments</u>** Cranberry Jelly/Sauce Hot Sauce (Low Sodium) Mint Jelly/Sauce Pepper Jelly Wasabi **<u>Condiments Higher Sodium</u>** **<u>(1 tbsp per day or less)</u>** Barbecue Sauce (Can use more if low sodium version) * Ketchup * Mustard Relish Tartar Sauce Worcestershire Sauce **<u>Sugar*</u>** Agave Syrup Brown Rice Syrup Corn Syrup^ Demerara Sugar Honey Icing Sugar Jam or Jelly Jet Puffed ® Marshmallow Crème Lemon Spread Maple Syrup^ Marmalade Marshmallow Fluff Molasses^

Vinaigrette and Marinade

Kuhne ®
Yogurt and Herbs
Yogurt and Garlic

Litehouse ®
Red Wine and Olive Oil
Vinaigrette
Raspberry Walnut
Vinaigrette

Marilyn's ®
Blackberry Blast
Classic Balsamic

President's Choice ® Blue
Menu™
Roasted Garlic and
Balsamic Vinaigrette
Pear and Walnut
Vinaigrette

Renee's Gourmet™
Poppy seed
Cucumber and Dill
Balsamic
Ravin' Raspberry

Rising Sun Farms®
Lemon Thyme
Pomegranate Balsamic
Fig Balsamic
Raspberry

Western Family ®
Raspberry Vinaigrette

Sugar (Brown, Cane, White,
Raw, Powdered, Coconut) *
Syrup

Low Sodium Snack Ideas
Carrot sticks and hummus
Celery and nut butter
Bell pepper strips
Cucumber slices
Apples and nut butter
Applesauce to-go pouches
Berries and plant-based
yogurt
Skinny pop popcorn
Roasted chickpea snacks
(higher in protein)
Roasted edamame (higher in
protein)
Snap pea crisps (higher in
protein)
Off the Eaten Path veggie
crisps
KIND bars
That's It fruit bars
Late July grain free lime and
sea salt tortilla chips
Purely Elizabeth Grain free
granola
MadeGood rice crispy
squares

WORKING WITH RENAL RECIPES: ADAPTING AND CUSTOMIZING FOR YOUR NEEDS

In this chapter, we explore the art of working with renal recipes to suit your personal preferences and meet your individual dietary restrictions. Renal recipes provide a foundation for creating delicious and kidney-friendly meals, but it's important to remember that they can be adapted and customized to cater to your specific needs. By learning strategies for modifying renal recipes, customizing them to meet your dietary restrictions, and adding variety and creativity, you can enjoy a wide range of satisfying and nourishing meals while supporting your kidney health.

STRATEGIES FOR MODIFYING RENAL RECIPES TO SUIT PERSONAL PREFERENCES

When it comes to modifying renal recipes to suit your personal preferences, there are several strategies you can employ to make the dishes more enjoyable and aligned with your taste buds. Here are some strategies for adapting renal recipes:

Adjust Flavors:

- Experiment with Herbs and Spices: Enhance the taste of renal recipes by experimenting with a variety of herbs, spices, and seasonings. These flavor enhancers can add depth and complexity to your dishes without relying on excessive salt or sodium.

- Use Low-Sodium Seasonings: Look for low-sodium alternatives to common seasonings such as soy sauce, Worcestershire sauce, or bouillon cubes. Opt for options labeled "low sodium" or "no salt added" to keep sodium levels in check while still adding flavor.

Swap Ingredients:

- Customize Protein Choices: If a renal recipe calls for a specific type of protein that you don't particularly enjoy or cannot consume due to dietary restrictions, consider swapping it with an alternative that suits your preferences. For example, if you prefer poultry over red meat, substitute chicken or turkey in place of beef in recipes like stews or stir-fries.

- Adapt Vegetables and Fruits: Modify the selection of vegetables and fruits used in recipes based on your preferences or seasonal availability. Explore a variety of options and experiment with different flavors and textures to keep the dishes interesting.

Modify Texture:

- Adjust Cooking Times: Adapt the cooking times to achieve the desired texture of ingredients. For example, if you prefer your vegetables to be crisp and retain some bite, reduce the cooking time slightly to prevent overcooking.

- Explore Different Cooking Methods: Experiment

with different cooking methods such as grilling, roasting, steaming, or stir-frying to achieve different textures and flavors. Each cooking technique can bring out unique characteristics of the ingredients and add variety to your meals.

- Blend or Puree Ingredients: If you prefer smoother textures, consider blending or pureeing certain ingredients to create creamy soups, sauces, or dips. This can be especially helpful for individuals with difficulty chewing or swallowing.

Adjust Seasoning Intensity:

- Taste and Adjust: As you prepare renal recipes, taste the dish along the way and make adjustments to the seasoning as needed. Start with less seasoning and gradually add more until you achieve the desired taste. This allows you to personalize the flavors to suit your preferences without compromising on the overall renal-friendly nature of the recipe.

CUSTOMIZING RECIPES TO MEET INDIVIDUAL DIETARY RESTRICTIONS

Customizing renal recipes to meet individual dietary restrictions is an essential aspect of creating a personalized kidney-friendly meal plan. Here are some strategies for customizing recipes based on common dietary restrictions:

Low-Sodium Diet:

- Reduce or Omit Salt: Adjust the amount of salt used in recipes or eliminate it altogether. Instead, enhance the flavors of your dishes with herbs, spices, citrus juices, vinegar, or low-sodium seasoning blends.

- Use Fresh Ingredients: Opt for fresh

ingredients whenever possible, as they generally contain lower sodium levels compared to canned or processed alternatives.

- Choose Low-Sodium Ingredients: Select low-sodium or sodium-free versions of condiments, sauces, broths, and canned goods to maintain strict control over your sodium intake.

Potassium and Phosphorus Restrictions:

- Select Low-Potassium Ingredients: Choose ingredients that are lower in potassium to manage your potassium intake. Examples include apples, berries, green beans, cauliflower, and white rice. Consult with your renal dietitian to determine specific potassium restrictions and recommended serving sizes.

- Limit High-Phosphorus Foods: If you have phosphorus restrictions, focus on reducing or avoiding high-phosphorus foods such as dairy products, nuts, seeds, chocolate, and processed meats. Opt for lower phosphorus alternatives and practice portion control.

- Leaching Technique: For certain high-potassium vegetables like potatoes or winter squash, you can reduce their potassium content by leaching. Soak the chopped or sliced vegetables in water for several hours before cooking to leach out some of the potassium.

Allergies or Food Intolerances:

- Identify Suitable Substitutes: If you have allergies or food intolerances, identify suitable substitutes for ingredients that trigger adverse reactions. For example, if you are lactose intolerant, use lactose-free dairy alternatives or explore non-dairy options like almond milk or coconut milk.

- Adjust Recipes Accordingly: Modify recipes by omitting or replacing allergenic ingredients with appropriate alternatives. Be mindful of cross-contamination and ensure that your cooking utensils and surfaces are thoroughly cleaned to avoid any potential allergen exposure.

Other Dietary Considerations:

- Gluten-Free Options: If you follow a gluten-free diet, opt for gluten-free grains like rice, quinoa, and gluten-free flours for baking. Check ingredient labels carefully to avoid hidden sources of gluten.

- Diabetes Management: If you have diabetes, work with your healthcare team and renal dietitian to adjust recipes to suit your blood sugar management goals. Focus on balancing carbohydrates, incorporating lean proteins, and choosing nutrient-dense, low-glycemic index foods.

TIPS FOR ADDING VARIETY AND CREATIVITY TO KIDNEY-FRIENDLY MEALS

Adding variety and creativity to your kidney-friendly meals is not only enjoyable but also important for maintaining a well-rounded and satisfying diet. Here are some detailed tips to help you infuse excitement and diversity into your kidney-friendly meals:

Experiment with Herbs, Spices, and Seasonings:

- Explore New Flavors: Incorporate a wide range of herbs, spices, and seasonings to add depth and complexity to your dishes. For example, try using cumin, turmeric, paprika, or smoked paprika to add rich flavors to your recipes. Experiment with different combinations and ratios to discover unique flavor profiles that appeal to your taste buds.

- Make Homemade Seasoning Blends: Create your own seasoning blends using a variety of herbs, spices, and salt-free seasonings. For example, you can mix garlic powder, onion powder, oregano, thyme, and black pepper to create an Italian-inspired seasoning blend. Customize the flavor profile of your meals while keeping sodium levels in check.

- Discover International Cuisine: Dive into the world of international cuisine and explore flavors from different cultures. Incorporate spices and herbs used in Mediterranean, Asian, Middle Eastern, or Latin American dishes to bring variety to your meals. For example, use garam masala, curry powder, or ginger in Indian-inspired dishes, or try using sesame oil and soy sauce for an Asian twist.

Try New Ingredients:

- Venture into Unfamiliar Produce: Expand your palate by trying new fruits, vegetables, and grains. Incorporate lesser-known varieties like jicama, bok choy, Swiss chard, farro, or freekeh to add a unique twist to your dishes. For example, use jicama as a crunchy addition to salads or try substituting traditional grains with farro in pilafs or salads for a nutty flavor.

- Explore Plant-Based Proteins: Incorporate plant-based protein sources such as tofu, tempeh, lentils, chickpeas, or black beans into your meals. These ingredients offer a wide range of flavors, textures, and cooking possibilities. For example, use chickpeas to make homemade hummus or blend silken tofu with herbs and spices to create a creamy dairy-free dressing.

- Incorporate Seasonal Produce: Embrace the flavors of each season by including seasonal fruits and vegetables in your meals. They not only provide freshness and variety but also tend to be more affordable and readily available. For example, in the summer, use fresh tomatoes, cucumbers, and basil to make a refreshing

Mediterranean-inspired salad or gazpacho.

Embrace Different Cooking Techniques:

- Grill or Roast: Experiment with grilling or roasting your proteins and vegetables for a delicious smoky flavor. This technique enhances the natural sweetness and adds a charred element to your dishes. For example, grill chicken skewers with a marinade of lemon, garlic, and herbs, or roast mixed vegetables with a sprinkle of olive oil, salt, and pepper for a caramelized flavor.

- Stir-Fry or Sauté: Stir-frying (my personal favorite) or sautéing allows for quick cooking and the combination of different flavors and textures. Mix a variety of vegetables, proteins, and seasonings for a colorful and flavorful meal. For example, stir-fry a medley of bell peppers, snap peas, tofu, and ginger with a splash of low-sodium soy sauce and sesame oil for a satisfying Asian-inspired dish.

- Use Fresh Herbs as Garnish: Add a vibrant touch to your dishes by garnishing them with fresh herbs like basil, cilantro, mint, or parsley. They not only enhance the presentation but also add aromatic flavors. For example, top a kidney-friendly lentil soup with a sprinkle of chopped fresh parsley or garnish a grilled vegetable salad with torn basil leaves.

Incorporate Texture and Color:

- Play with Textures: Combine different textures in your meals to create a more exciting eating experience. Mix crispy vegetables like bell peppers or cucumbers with tender proteins like grilled chicken or flaked fish, or incorporate crunchy toppings like toasted nuts or seeds for added texture. For example, add toasted almond slices to a kidney-friendly quinoa salad or sprinkle crushed walnuts on top of roasted vegetables.

- Add Colorful Ingredients: Opt for a variety

of colorful fruits and vegetables to make your meals visually appealing. The vibrant hues not only make the dishes more enticing but also provide a diverse array of nutrients. For example, add sliced strawberries or pomegranate arils to a spinach salad or include roasted beets for a pop of color in grain bowls.

Modify Cooking Methods and Presentation:

- Explore Different Culinary Techniques: Try new cooking methods like steaming, braising, or poaching to bring out different flavors and textures in your ingredients. For example, steam asparagus until tender-crisp, braise chicken with tomatoes and herbs for a rich and tender dish, or poach delicate fish in a flavorful broth.

- Experiment with Plating: Enhance the dining experience by paying attention to how you present your meals. Experiment with different plating techniques to make your dishes visually appealing and appetizing. For example, arrange colorful grilled vegetables in a visually appealing pattern on a plate or use a piping bag to create attractive swirls of mashed sweet potatoes.

Remember, variety and creativity are key to keeping your kidney-friendly meals interesting and enjoyable. Don't be afraid to step out of your comfort zone and try new ingredients, flavors, and cooking techniques.

WORKING WITH A DIETITIAN: PERSONALIZED GUIDANCE FOR OPTIMAL HEALTH

In this chapter, we will explore the vital role of a renal dietitian in managing kidney disease and discuss the benefits of collaborating with a dietitian to develop a customized meal plan. We will also provide guidance on finding a renal dietitian and highlight the advantages of ongoing support from a healthcare professional. Let's delve into the world of renal dietetics and discover how it can empower you on your kidney health journey.

THE ROLE OF A RENAL DIETITIAN IN MANAGING KIDNEY DISEASE

A renal dietitian is a specialized healthcare professional who focuses on providing dietary guidance and support for individuals with kidney disease. They possess in-depth knowledge of the unique nutritional needs and challenges faced by those with kidney disease.

Compared to traditional dietitians, renal dietitians have specific expertise in managing kidney disease and its associated complications. They are trained to interpret lab results, assess dietary needs based on individual kidney function and other health parameters, and develop personalized meal plans tailored to each person's unique requirements.

Renal dietitians play a crucial role in educating individuals about kidney-friendly foods, managing nutrient intake, and making appropriate dietary modifications to slow the progression of kidney disease and reduce the risk of complications. They work closely with other members of the healthcare team to provide comprehensive care and support.

COLLABORATING WITH A DIETITIAN TO DEVELOP A CUSTOMIZED MEAL PLAN

Collaborating with a renal dietitian to develop a customized meal plan is a key aspect of effectively managing kidney disease and achieving optimal health outcomes. This collaborative approach ensures that your dietary recommendations are tailored to your unique needs, preferences, and medical condition. Let's explore the benefits and process of collaborating with a dietitian to develop a customized meal plan:

Individualized Assessment:

A renal dietitian will conduct a thorough assessment of your health, medical history, kidney function, and nutritional needs. They will take into consideration factors such as your age, weight, activity level, medications, and underlying health conditions. This assessment provides a comprehensive understanding of your specific nutritional requirements and any potential dietary restrictions.

Personalized Goals and Preferences:

During the collaboration, the dietitian will work with you to establish personalized goals based on your specific needs and preferences. These goals may include managing blood pressure, controlling blood sugar levels, maintaining an appropriate weight, or optimizing nutrient intake. Your preferences, cultural background, and culinary preferences will also be taken into account to ensure that your meal plan is enjoyable and sustainable.

Customized Meal Planning:

Based on the assessment and goals, the dietitian will develop a customized meal plan that meets your unique nutritional needs. The meal plan will specify portion sizes, food choices, and nutrient distribution throughout the day. It will focus on kidney-friendly foods while considering factors such as sodium, phosphorus, potassium, protein, and fluid intake. The dietitian will educate you on food substitutions, label reading, and cooking techniques to help you navigate grocery shopping and meal preparation effectively.

Education and Guidance:

Collaborating with a dietitian provides you with valuable education and guidance on kidney nutrition. The dietitian will explain the role of various nutrients in kidney health and provide recommendations on managing sodium, phosphorus, potassium, and protein intake. They will address any questions or concerns you may have and help you understand how your dietary choices can impact your kidney function. By gaining knowledge and understanding, you will be empowered to make informed decisions about your food choices.

Ongoing Support and Monitoring:

Once your customized meal plan is in place, the dietitian will provide ongoing support and monitoring. Regular follow-up appointments will allow the dietitian to track your progress, review your lab results, and make any necessary adjustments to your meal plan. They will provide ongoing guidance and support to help you overcome any challenges and maintain adherence to your dietary recommendations.

Collaborating with a dietitian to develop a customized meal plan ensures that your nutritional needs are addressed comprehensively. By working together, you can create a meal plan that is practical, enjoyable, and tailored to your individual circumstances. The dietitian's expertise in kidney nutrition allows them to consider specific dietary requirements, restrictions, and potential interactions with medications to develop a meal plan that supports your kidney health and overall well-being.

Remember, the meal plan is not a one-size-fits-all approach. It is a dynamic tool that can be adjusted based on your changing needs, preferences, and medical condition. The collaboration with a dietitian provides ongoing support and guidance, helping you navigate the challenges of managing kidney disease while enjoying a varied and balanced diet.

HOW TO FIND A RENAL DIETITIAN

Finding a renal dietitian to support your kidney health journey is an important step in managing kidney disease effectively. Renal dietitians are specialized professionals with expertise in kidney nutrition, and their guidance can be invaluable in developing a personalized meal plan and providing ongoing support. Here are some tips to help you find a renal dietitian:

Consult Your Healthcare Team:

Start by consulting your healthcare team, including your nephrologist or primary care physician. They can provide recommendations and referrals to renal dietitians in your area. Your healthcare team is familiar with your specific medical condition and can guide you in finding a dietitian who specializes in kidney health.

Local Medical Centers and Hospitals:

Contact local medical centers, hospitals, or dialysis centers in your area. These institutions often have renal dietitians as part of their healthcare team. Reach out to their nutrition departments or ask your healthcare provider for information on dietitians who specialize in kidney nutrition.

Online Directories and Professional Organizations:

Check online directories and professional organizations that specialize in kidney health and nutrition. Websites like the Academy of Nutrition and Dietetics and the National Kidney Foundation often have directories of registered dietitians who specialize in kidney nutrition. You can search for dietitians in your area or access online consultations if in-person options are limited.

Kidney Support Groups and Communities:

Join kidney support groups or communities where individuals with kidney disease gather to share experiences and information. These groups may have recommendations or firsthand experiences with renal dietitians who have helped them in their journey. Engaging with these communities can provide valuable insights and recommendations on finding a renal dietitian.

Reputable Online Resources:

Explore reputable online platforms that connect individuals with specialized renal dietitians. Platforms such as Plant-Powered Kidneys, led by Jen Hernandez, and Kidney Nutrition Institute, led by Jessianna Saville, are highly recommended resources. These platforms work closely with Dadvice TV, providing educational content and access to reputable renal dietitians. They offer online consultations and guidance, ensuring that you can connect with qualified renal dietitians regardless of your location.

When selecting a renal dietitian, consider their experience, credentials, and expertise in kidney nutrition. Look for registered dietitians who have specialized training or certifications in renal nutrition. Take the time to schedule an initial consultation to assess their approach, communication style, and compatibility with your needs.

Remember, finding a renal dietitian is an investment in your health and well-being. Their specialized knowledge and guidance can help you navigate the complexities of managing kidney disease through nutrition. Working closely with a renal dietitian ensures that your dietary recommendations are tailored to your specific needs, promotes better adherence to your meal plan, and enhances your overall health outcomes.

BENEFITS OF ONGOING SUPPORT AND GUIDANCE FROM A HEALTHCARE PROFESSIONAL

Ongoing support from a renal dietitian can significantly impact your kidney health journey. Benefits include:

Personalized Approach: A renal dietitian provides personalized guidance based on your specific needs, helping you navigate the complexities of managing kidney disease through nutrition.

Expertise in Kidney Health: Renal dietitians have specialized knowledge and experience in managing kidney disease and its unique dietary considerations. They stay updated on the latest research and guidelines in renal nutrition, ensuring you receive accurate and evidence-based information.

Monitoring and Adjustments: Regular follow-up appointments with a dietitian allow for ongoing monitoring of your progress, lab results, and dietary adherence. This helps identify any necessary adjustments to your meal plan and ensures that it remains aligned with your changing health needs.

Education and Empowerment: Dietitians provide education on kidney-friendly foods, portion control, label reading, and strategies for managing dietary challenges. This knowledge empowers you to make informed choices, fostering independence and self-management of your diet.

Emotional Support: Managing kidney disease can be overwhelming, and a dietitian can provide emotional support and motivation. They understand the challenges you face and can offer guidance to help you overcome dietary obstacles while maintaining a positive mindset.

Collaboration with Healthcare Team: Renal dietitians work collaboratively with your healthcare team, including nephrologists, nurses, and other specialists. They ensure seamless communication, helping to optimize your overall care and treatment outcomes.

By working with a renal dietitian, you gain access to specialized expertise and personalized guidance, empowering you to make informed choices about your nutrition and effectively manage kidney disease.

PLANT-BASED PROTEIN POWER: MAXIMIZING NUTRITION WITH PLANT PROTEINS

In this chapter, we delve into the world of plant-based protein sources and their significant role in supporting a kidney-friendly diet. We will explore the benefits of plant-based protein sources, discuss their nutritional value, health advantages, and provide guidance on incorporating these protein-rich options into your meals. By embracing plant-based proteins, you can optimize your nutrition while promoting kidney health and overall well-being.

EXPLORING THE BENEFITS OF PLANT-BASED PROTEIN SOURCES

Comprehensive Nutrition: Plant-based protein sources provide a wealth of essential nutrients, making them an excellent choice for a well-rounded and nourishing diet. These protein sources are not only rich in protein but also contain an array of vitamins, minerals, antioxidants, and dietary fiber.

The combination of these nutrients supports overall health, strengthens the immune system, and promotes optimal organ function.

Lower Saturated Fat: Compared to animal-based protein sources, plant proteins are generally lower in saturated fat. This is beneficial for kidney health, as a diet low in saturated fat helps to reduce the risk of heart disease, high blood pressure, and other cardiovascular complications. By incorporating more plant-based protein into your diet, you can support both kidney health and cardiovascular well-being.

Rich in Fiber: Plant-based protein sources are often accompanied by dietary fiber, which offers multiple benefits for kidney health. Fiber aids in maintaining regular bowel movements and preventing constipation, a common concern for individuals with kidney disease. Additionally, dietary fiber helps to stabilize blood sugar levels, promote satiety, and support weight management. By choosing plant-based protein sources, you can effortlessly increase your fiber intake and promote digestive health.

Antioxidant Power: Many plant-based protein sources are packed with antioxidants, which are beneficial compounds that protect cells from damage caused by harmful free radicals. These antioxidants help to reduce inflammation, prevent oxidative stress, and support the overall health of your kidneys. By incorporating plant-based protein sources rich in antioxidants, such as fruits, vegetables, legumes, nuts, and seeds, you can promote kidney health and reduce the risk of chronic diseases.

Reduced Acid Load and Phosphorus Control: Plant proteins have a lower acid load compared to animal proteins. This means that when you consume plant-based proteins, your body produces fewer acidic byproducts during digestion. This is particularly advantageous for individuals with kidney disease, as it helps to maintain a healthier acid-base balance and reduce the strain on the kidneys. Additionally, plant proteins have a lower phosphorus content compared to certain animal proteins, which is crucial for individuals with kidney disease who need to manage their phosphorus levels.

Allergy-Friendly and Digestive Benefits: Plant-based protein sources are often hypoallergenic, making them suitable for individuals with allergies or sensitivities to animal proteins. Moreover, plant proteins tend to be easier to digest, as they do not contain complex animal fats and are typically accompanied by dietary fiber. This can alleviate digestive discomfort and provide relief for individuals with gastrointestinal issues.

By exploring the benefits of plant-based protein sources, you can make informed choices that support kidney health and overall well-being. Incorporating a variety of plant proteins into your diet not only ensures adequate protein intake but also enhances the nutritional profile of your meals.

NUTRITIONAL VALUE AND HEALTH ADVANTAGES OF PLANT PROTEINS

Balanced Amino Acid Profile: Plant proteins, although often considered incomplete proteins individually, can be combined to create a complete amino acid profile. By incorporating a variety of plant-based protein sources into your diet, such as legumes, whole grains, nuts, and seeds, you can obtain all the essential amino acids your body needs for optimal health. This ensures that you receive a balanced and diverse array of amino acids to support various bodily functions, including muscle repair, immune function, and hormone production.

Kidney Health Benefits: Plant proteins offer unique advantages for kidney health compared to animal proteins. Plant-based protein sources have a lower acid load, meaning they produce fewer acidic byproducts during digestion. This is important because excessive acid production can place a burden on the kidneys and potentially contribute to the progression of kidney disease. By choosing plant proteins, you can help maintain a healthier acid-base balance and alleviate stress on the kidneys.

Cardiovascular Support: Plant proteins are generally lower in saturated fat and cholesterol compared to animal proteins. High consumption of saturated fat and cholesterol has been linked to an increased risk of heart disease and other cardiovascular complications. By incorporating more plant-based proteins into your diet, you can support heart health and reduce the risk of cardiovascular diseases commonly associated with kidney disease.

Rich in Fiber: Plant proteins are often accompanied by dietary fiber, which is important for maintaining healthy digestion and preventing constipation. Fiber adds bulk to the diet, promotes regular bowel movements, and supports gastrointestinal health. By choosing plant proteins, you can increase your fiber intake and promote optimal digestive function, which is particularly beneficial for individuals with kidney disease who may experience digestive challenges.

Antioxidant and Anti-inflammatory Properties: Many plant-based protein sources, such as legumes, nuts, seeds, and colorful fruits and vegetables, are rich in antioxidants and anti-inflammatory compounds. These nutrients help combat oxidative stress, reduce inflammation, and protect against chronic diseases, including kidney disease. By incorporating plant proteins with high antioxidant content, you can support kidney health and mitigate the damaging effects of free radicals and inflammation.

Lower Phosphorus Content: Certain plant-based protein sources, such as legumes and some whole grains, have a lower phosphorus content compared to animal proteins. This is particularly advantageous for individuals with kidney disease who need to manage their phosphorus levels. By incorporating more plant proteins into your diet, you can help control phosphorus intake and support kidney health.

INCORPORATING PLANT-BASED PROTEINS INTO A KIDNEY-FRIENDLY DIET

Diverse Protein Sources: Embrace the wide array of plant-based protein sources available to you. Include a variety of legumes such as beans (black beans, kidney beans, chickpeas), lentils, and split peas. Incorporate whole grains like quinoa, brown rice, and oats, which provide not only protein but also fiber and essential nutrients. Explore plant-based protein options like tofu, tempeh, edamame, and seitan. Additionally, nuts and seeds such as almonds, walnuts, chia seeds, and hemp seeds can be excellent sources of protein and healthy fats.

Balanced Meals: Create well-balanced meals by combining plant-based proteins with other kidney-friendly components. Pair plant proteins with whole grains like quinoa or brown rice, which provide complementary amino acids and additional nutrients. Add a variety of vegetables, both cooked and raw, to provide a range of vitamins, minerals, and fiber. Consider incorporating plant-based proteins into soups, stews, salads, stir-fries, and grain bowls for a satisfying and nutrient-packed meal.

Recipe Adaptation: Modify traditional recipes to feature plant-based proteins instead of animal proteins. For example, replace ground meat with cooked lentils or beans in dishes like chili, tacos, or pasta sauces. Use tofu or tempeh as a substitute for meat in stir-fries, curries, or kebabs. Experiment with plant-based burgers made from legumes, grains, or vegetables. By adapting recipes, you can enjoy familiar flavors and textures while incorporating plant-based proteins into your meals.

Snack Options: Incorporate plant-based protein snacks into your daily routine. Enjoy a handful of mixed nuts or seeds as a nutritious snack. Opt for hummus made from chickpeas or other legumes and pair it with fresh vegetables for a satisfying and protein-rich dip. Explore plant-based protein bars or homemade energy balls made from dates, nuts, and seeds for a convenient on-the-go snack.

Recipe Resources: Explore cookbooks, online resources, and reputable websites that specialize in plant-based recipes for kidney health. Look for recipes that specifically mention their suitability for individuals with kidney disease or those that are low in potassium, phosphorus, and sodium. Platforms like Plant-Powered Kidneys, Kidney Nutrition Institute, and Dadvice TV often feature plant-based recipes and resources designed for kidney health.

Professional Guidance: Consult with your renal dietitian to receive personalized guidance on incorporating plant-based proteins into your kidney-friendly diet. They can help you create a meal plan that suits your dietary restrictions, preferences, and nutritional needs. A renal dietitian can also provide tips on portion sizes, cooking methods, and proper meal timing to ensure you meet your protein requirements while supporting your kidney health.

As you conclude this chapter, I encourage you to embark on an exciting journey of integrating more plant-based foods into your kidney-friendly diet. Plant-based proteins offer a multitude of health benefits, from their balanced amino acid profiles to their rich array of nutrients and potential advantages for kidney health. By incorporating plant-based proteins into your meals, you can enjoy the nutritional power they bring while supporting your overall well-being.

Take small steps at first, gradually introducing new plant-based protein sources and experimenting with creative recipes. Begin by swapping out animal proteins with plant-based alternatives in a few meals each week. Embrace the diversity of legumes, whole grains, nuts, seeds, and plant-based protein options available to you, and discover the flavors and textures they bring to your plate.

Remember, you don't have to completely eliminate animal proteins if you enjoy them. It's about finding a balance that suits your individual needs and preferences. By incorporating more plant-based proteins, you can increase your intake of vital nutrients, fiber, and antioxidants, while potentially reducing the strain on your kidneys and supporting better overall health.

Consult with your renal dietitian, explore reputable resources, and connect with communities like Plant-Powered Kidneys,

Kidney Nutrition Institute, and Dadvice TV for inspiration and guidance. They can provide valuable insights, recipes, and tips tailored to individuals with kidney disease, helping you navigate your plant-based journey with confidence.

By embracing plant-based proteins, you are not only nourishing your body but also contributing to a more sustainable and environmentally friendly food system. Your choices can make a positive impact on your health, the planet, and the lives of animals.

So, start today and explore the abundance of delicious plant-based protein options waiting to be discovered. Your kidney-friendly diet will be enriched with new flavors, textures, and nutritional benefits, paving the way for a healthier and more vibrant life.

PLANT-BASED BENEFITS: CHOOSING PLANT SOURCES OVER ANIMAL SOURCES

In this chapter, we will explore the advantages of incorporating plant-based foods into a kidney-friendly diet. We'll discuss the benefits of plant-based protein sources compared to animal sources and provide practical tips for incorporating plant-based meals into your routine. Additionally, we'll highlight the versatility of soy as a valuable plant-based protein option for individuals with kidney disease.

EXPLORING THE ADVANTAGES OF PLANT-BASED FOODS FOR KIDNEY HEALTH

Incorporating plant-based foods into a kidney-friendly diet offers several advantages that can support overall kidney health. Let's dive deeper into the benefits of plant-based foods for individuals with kidney disease:

Lower Sodium Content:

Plant-based foods, such as fruits, vegetables, legumes, and whole grains, are naturally low in sodium. High sodium intake can lead to fluid retention, increased blood pressure, and strain on the kidneys. By choosing plant-based options, you can reduce your sodium intake and better manage blood pressure, thus supporting kidney function and overall cardiovascular health.

Reduced Phosphorus Load:

Many animal-based foods, such as meat, dairy products, and processed foods, tend to be high in phosphorus. For individuals with kidney disease, managing phosphorus levels is crucial, as excessive phosphorus intake can lead to mineral imbalances, bone issues, and complications related to kidney function. Plant-based protein sources, such as legumes, tofu, and whole grains, generally have lower phosphorus content, making them kidney-friendly choices that can help maintain a balance in phosphorus levels.

Heart-Healthy Fats:

Plant-based foods are often rich in heart-healthy fats, such as monounsaturated and polyunsaturated fats. These fats can help lower cholesterol levels, reduce inflammation, and promote cardiovascular health. By incorporating sources like avocados, nuts, seeds, and olive oil into your diet, you can support heart health while reducing the risk of cardiovascular complications commonly associated with kidney disease.

Higher Fiber Content:

Plant-based foods are typically high in dietary fiber, which offers numerous health benefits. Fiber helps regulate blood sugar levels, promotes digestive health, and contributes to satiety and weight management. Additionally, soluble fiber can help lower cholesterol levels, which is especially important for individuals with kidney disease who are at higher risk for cardiovascular issues.

Abundance of Phytonutrients and Antioxidants:

Plant-based foods are rich in phytonutrients and antioxidants, which have been shown to have protective effects against chronic diseases, including kidney disease. These compounds help reduce inflammation, neutralize harmful free radicals, and support overall cellular health. Fruits, vegetables, herbs, and spices offer a wide range of these beneficial compounds, providing an array of flavors, colors, and health-promoting properties.

PLANT-BASED PROTEIN SOURCES AND THEIR BENEFITS OVER ANIMAL SOURCES

When it comes to protein intake for individuals with kidney disease, plant-based protein sources offer several advantages over animal sources. Let's explore the benefits of incorporating plant-based protein into your diet:

Reduced Phosphorus Content:

Plant-based protein sources generally have lower phosphorus content compared to animal-based protein sources. This is significant for individuals with kidney disease, as high phosphorus levels can be detrimental to kidney health and bone health. By choosing plant-based proteins like legumes, tofu, and seitan, you can help maintain a better balance of phosphorus in your diet, reducing the strain on your kidneys and supporting overall kidney health.

Lower Sodium Content:

Plant-based protein sources are typically lower in sodium compared to animal-based proteins. High sodium intake can lead to fluid retention and increased blood pressure, which can worsen kidney function. By selecting plant-based proteins such as lentils, quinoa, and tempeh, you can limit your sodium intake and better manage blood pressure, reducing the risk of complications associated with kidney disease.

Heart-Healthy Fats:

Many plant-based protein sources are rich in heart-healthy fats, such as monounsaturated and polyunsaturated fats. These fats can help lower cholesterol levels, reduce inflammation, and improve cardiovascular health. By incorporating plant-based proteins like nuts, seeds, and avocados into your diet, you can support heart health and decrease the risk of cardiovascular complications, which are common in individuals with kidney disease.

Fiber and Nutrient Content:

Plant-based protein sources often come bundled with additional fiber, vitamins, minerals, and phytonutrients. Fiber helps regulate blood sugar levels, promotes digestive health, and contributes to satiety and weight management. Fruits, vegetables, whole grains, legumes, nuts, and seeds are excellent sources of plant-based protein that provide a wide range of nutrients, supporting overall health and well-being.

Lower Saturated Fat and Cholesterol:

Animal-based protein sources, such as red meat, poultry, and dairy products, can be high in saturated fat and cholesterol. Excessive intake of saturated fat and cholesterol can contribute to heart disease, a common concern for individuals with kidney disease. By opting for plant-based protein sources, you can reduce your saturated fat and cholesterol intake, supporting cardiovascular health and minimizing the risk of related complications.

Reduced Risk of Hyperfiltration:

Hyperfiltration refers to an increased blood flow through the kidneys, which can put additional stress on these organs. Animal-based protein sources have been associated with higher levels of protein waste products in the blood, leading to increased glomerular filtration rate (GFR) and potential hyperfiltration. Plant-based protein sources, on the other hand, tend to have a more favorable impact on GFR, reducing the risk of hyperfiltration and potential kidney damage.

Balanced pH Levels:

Plant-based protein sources have the advantage of promoting a more alkaline environment in the body. Animal-based proteins, particularly sulfur-containing amino acids found in meat and dairy, have been associated with the production of acid byproducts during metabolism. This can lead to a more acidic pH balance in the body, which may contribute to kidney stone formation and calcium loss from bones. Plant-based proteins, being generally lower in sulfur-containing amino acids, have a more neutralizing effect on pH levels and can help maintain a healthier acid-base balance.

Environmental Sustainability:

Choosing plant-based protein sources can also have positive impacts on the environment. Animal agriculture is resource-intensive and contributes to greenhouse gas emissions. By incorporating more plant-based proteins into your diet, you can contribute to sustainable food choices and reduce your carbon footprint.

INCORPORATING PLANT-BASED MEALS INTO A KIDNEY-FRIENDLY DIET

Adding plant-based meals to your kidney-friendly diet can provide numerous health benefits while adding variety and flavor to your meals. Here are some tips to help you successfully incorporate plant-based meals into your routine:

Emphasize Whole Foods:

Focus on incorporating whole plant-based foods such as fruits, vegetables, whole grains, legumes, nuts, and seeds into your meals. These foods are rich in fiber, vitamins, minerals, and phytonutrients that support overall health and kidney function.

Explore New Flavors and Cuisines:

Experiment with different herbs, spices, and seasonings to add flavor and depth to your plant-based meals. This can make your dishes more exciting and satisfying. Try incorporating global cuisines that naturally include plant-based meals, such as Mediterranean, Asian, or Middle Eastern cuisines.

Optimize Plant-Based Protein Sources:

Include a variety of plant-based protein sources in your meals to ensure you meet your protein needs. Legumes, such as lentils, chickpeas, and beans, are excellent sources of plant-based protein. Tofu, tempeh, and seitan are other versatile options. Incorporate these proteins into stir-fries, salads, soups, or grain bowls.

Explore Whole Grains:

Introduce a variety of whole grains into your diet, such as quinoa, brown rice, bulgur, farro, or whole wheat pasta. These grains provide additional nutrients and fiber to your meals. Use them as a base for salads, side dishes, or main courses.

Get Creative with Vegetables:

Make vegetables the star of your plant-based meals by exploring different cooking methods and preparations. Roast vegetables with herbs and spices, sauté them with garlic and olive oil, or grill them to enhance their natural flavors. Consider incorporating a wide range of colorful vegetables to ensure a diverse nutrient profile.

Include Healthy Fats:

Incorporate plant-based fats into your meals, such as avocados, nuts, seeds, and olive oil. These healthy fats provide essential fatty acids and can enhance the flavor and satiety of your plant-based dishes. Use them in salad dressings, as toppings, or for sautéing vegetables.

Adapt Your Favorite Recipes:

Modify your favorite recipes to make them plant-based. Replace animal-based proteins with plant-based alternatives, such as using lentils or tofu instead of meat. Experiment with different combinations of vegetables, grains, and legumes to create delicious and satisfying plant-based versions of your favorite meals.

Plan Ahead:

Take the time to plan your plant-based meals in advance. This will help you ensure that you have the necessary ingredients on hand and make it easier to stick to your dietary goals. Consider batch cooking and meal prepping to save time during busy days.

THE VERSATILITY OF SOY

Soy is a versatile plant-based protein source that offers a multitude of benefits for individuals with kidney disease. Let's explore the versatility of soy and how it can be incorporated into a kidney-friendly diet:

Tofu: Tofu, also known as bean curd, is a popular soy product with a mild taste and a versatile texture. It is made by coagulating soy milk and pressing it into solid blocks. Tofu comes in various firmness levels, including soft, medium, and firm, each with its own unique culinary uses. It readily absorbs the flavors of marinades, spices, and sauces, making it an excellent addition to stir-fries, curries, soups, and salads. It can be grilled, pan-fried, or even blended into smoothies or desserts for added protein and creaminess.

Tempeh: Tempeh is a fermented soybean product that has a slightly nutty flavor and a firm texture. It is made by fermenting cooked soybeans with a specific type of fungus. Tempeh is rich in protein, fiber, and probiotics, which can support digestive health. It can be marinated, crumbled, or sliced and used in a variety of dishes such as stir-fries, sandwiches, wraps, or as a topping for salads. Its unique texture and savory taste make it a popular choice for those looking for a plant-based protein alternative.

Edamame: Edamame refers to young, green soybeans that are harvested before they fully mature. They are commonly found in the pod and are usually boiled or steamed before consumption. Edamame is a nutritious and convenient snack that can be enjoyed on its own, sprinkled with a touch of salt, or added to salads, stir-fries, soups, or grain bowls. They provide a good source of plant-based protein, fiber, vitamins, and minerals.

Soy Milk: Soy milk is a plant-based milk alternative made from soaked and ground soybeans. It is an excellent option for individuals who are lactose intolerant or following a vegan lifestyle. Soy milk can be used as a dairy milk substitute in various recipes, including smoothies, cereal, baked goods, and savory dishes. Opt for unsweetened varieties to keep the sugar content in check.

Soy Yogurt and Cheese: Soy-based yogurt and cheese alternatives are available for individuals seeking dairy-free options. These products offer a similar taste and texture to their dairy counterparts and can be enjoyed as a snack, used in recipes, or added to smoothies.

The versatility of soy lies not only in its various forms but also in its ability to blend seamlessly into a wide range of cuisines and recipes. Whether you are creating Asian-inspired stir-fries, hearty vegetarian burgers, creamy smoothies, or wholesome salads, soy can be a valuable ingredient that provides plant-based protein and enhances the taste and texture of your dishes.

When incorporating soy into your kidney-friendly diet, it is essential to choose low-sodium options and pay attention to portion sizes. Consult with your renal dietitian to determine the appropriate serving size and frequency of soy-based products based on your specific dietary needs and medical condition.

UNDERSTANDING PRAL (POTENTIAL RENAL ACID LOAD)

Maintaining a balanced acid-base environment is crucial for overall health, and especially important for individuals with kidney disease. The kidneys play a vital role in regulating acid-base balance by filtering and excreting waste products and maintaining optimal pH levels in the body. When acid-base balance is disrupted, it can put a strain on the kidneys and potentially worsen kidney function.

In this chapter, we will explore the concept of PRAL (Potential Renal Acid Load) as a measure of a food's impact on acid-base balance. While the topic may seem technical at first, I will do my best to break it down into easily understandable terms. Understanding PRAL can provide valuable insights into optimizing the kidney-friendly diet and promoting better kidney health. If you PRAL confuses you, don't worry – a Renal Dietitian will be an expert at PRAL!

PRAL is a method used to assess the acidifying or alkalizing potential of foods on the body. It measures the net acid load that a specific food will have on the kidneys after it is metabolized. By calculating PRAL values, we can categorize foods as either acid-forming or alkaline-forming based on their impact on the body's acid-base balance.

HOW UNDERSTANDING PRAL CAN HELP OPTIMIZE THE KIDNEY-FRIENDLY DIET

PRAL values can be valuable tools for individuals with kidney disease to tailor their diet and make informed food choices. By incorporating foods with lower PRAL values, we can help maintain a more balanced acid-base environment in the body, reducing the strain on the kidneys. Optimizing the kidney-friendly diet with PRAL awareness can support overall kidney health and potentially slow the progression of kidney disease.

Understanding the PRAL values of different foods empowers individuals to make conscious decisions that promote a healthier acid-base balance. It allows for a more personalized approach to the kidney-friendly diet, as it takes into account the specific needs and challenges of each individual's kidney health.

By considering PRAL values, individuals can choose foods that have a lower acid load and are more alkaline-forming, which can help offset the acid-forming effects of certain foods. This knowledge can assist in meal planning, food selection, and creating a balanced diet that supports kidney health.

What is PRAL?

PRAL is a measure used to assess the acidifying or alkalizing potential of foods on the body. It helps us understand how different foods affect the acid-base balance in our bodies, particularly in relation to kidney health. PRAL takes into account the composition of foods and their impact on the acidity or alkalinity of our internal environment.

PRAL is based on the premise that when certain foods are metabolized, they can generate either acidic or alkaline byproducts. These byproducts can influence the pH balance in our body fluids, including the blood and urine. By understanding the PRAL values of foods, we can make informed choices to promote a more balanced acid-base environment.

How PRAL is Calculated and Expressed

PRAL values are calculated by analyzing the content of potential acid or base-forming components in a food item. These components include minerals such as potassium, calcium, magnesium, and phosphorus, as well as proteins and other nutrients. The values are assigned based on the potential acid or base load generated during the metabolic breakdown of these components.

PRAL values are expressed in milliequivalents (mEq) per 100 grams (g) or milliequivalents per serving size of a food. The values can be positive, indicating an acid-forming potential, or negative, suggesting an alkaline-forming potential. The higher the positive PRAL value, the greater the acid-forming potential of the food, while the lower the negative value, the more alkaline-forming it is.

The Role of Acid-forming and Alkaline-forming Foods in PRAL

Different foods have varying effects on the acid-base balance in our bodies. Acid-forming foods tend to contain higher amounts of certain minerals, such as sulfur and phosphorus, and can increase the acid load in our system. Examples of acid-forming foods include animal protein, processed foods, refined grains, and certain beverages.

On the other hand, alkaline-forming foods have the potential to help neutralize excess acids and promote a more balanced internal environment. These foods often contain higher amounts of alkalizing minerals, such as potassium, calcium, and magnesium. Examples of alkaline-forming foods include fruits, vegetables, legumes, and certain nuts and seeds.

By understanding the role of acid-forming and alkaline-forming foods in PRAL, we can make conscious choices to include a greater proportion of alkaline-forming foods in our diet. This can help counterbalance the acid load from other dietary sources and promote a healthier acid-base balance.

THE IMPORTANCE OF MAINTAINING A BALANCED ACID-BASE ENVIRONMENT IN THE BODY

Maintaining a balanced acid-base environment is crucial for optimal health and well-being. The body operates within a narrow pH range, and any significant deviations can disrupt normal physiological processes. The acid-base balance affects various systems in the body, including enzyme activity, cellular function, hormone regulation, and the functioning of organs such as the kidneys.

The acid-base balance is measured using the pH scale, which ranges from 0 to 14. A pH of 7 is considered neutral, while values below 7 indicate acidity and values above 7 indicate alkalinity. The body's blood pH is tightly regulated around a slightly alkaline level of 7.35 to 7.45.

An imbalance in the acid-base environment can lead to acidosis or alkalosis. Acidosis occurs when there is an excess of acid or a decrease in the bicarbonate levels in the blood, resulting in a decrease in pH. This can happen due to factors such as metabolic disorders, respiratory conditions, or excessive production of acids through processes like uncontrolled diabetes or intense exercise. Alkalosis, on the other hand, occurs when there is an excess of alkaline substances or an increase in bicarbonate levels, leading to an increase in pH. This can be caused by factors such as prolonged vomiting, certain medications, or underlying metabolic conditions.

The Role of the Kidneys in Regulating Acid-Base Balance

The kidneys play a pivotal role in maintaining acid-base balance through various mechanisms. They help regulate the levels of bicarbonate ions (HCO_3-) in the blood, which act as a buffer to neutralize excess acids. The kidneys filter blood and selectively reabsorb or excrete certain substances to maintain a stable pH.

When the body experiences acidosis, the kidneys increase the excretion of hydrogen ions ($H+$) and generate bicarbonate ions (HCO_3-) to restore balance. The hydrogen ions are combined with ammonia (NH_3) to form ammonium (NH_4+), which can be excreted in the urine. The kidneys also reabsorb bicarbonate ions from the urine back into the bloodstream to replenish the bicarbonate buffer.

Conversely, in the case of alkalosis, the kidneys decrease hydrogen ion excretion and reduce bicarbonate reabsorption. This helps to conserve hydrogen ions and excrete excess bicarbonate ions, thus restoring acid-base balance.

The Potential Consequences of Prolonged Acidosis or Alkalosis on Kidney Health

Prolonged acidosis or alkalosis can have detrimental effects on kidney health. Acidosis can lead to the formation of kidney stones, as the increased acidity promotes the crystallization of certain minerals in the urine. This can cause blockages in the urinary tract and potentially damage the kidneys. Additionally, acidosis can contribute to the development and progression of chronic kidney disease by impairing kidney function over time. The prolonged presence of excess acid in the body can cause inflammation and damage to the delicate structures of the kidneys.

Alkalosis, although less common than acidosis, can also impact kidney health. It can interfere with the kidney's ability to reabsorb certain electrolytes, such as calcium and magnesium, leading to imbalances and potentially affecting overall kidney function. Additionally, alkalosis can disrupt the normal filtration and reabsorption processes in the kidneys, impairing their ability to maintain proper fluid and electrolyte balance.

It is important to note that while diet plays a role in acid-base balance, other factors, such as respiratory function and certain medical conditions, also contribute to maintaining the balance. However, making dietary choices that promote a balanced acid-base environment can support kidney health and overall well-being.

Understanding Acid-Forming Foods and Their Impact on PRAL

Acid-forming foods are those that, when metabolized by the body, leave behind acidic residue or byproducts. These residues can affect the body's acid-base balance and contribute to an increased acid load. The PRAL is a measure that quantifies the acid or alkaline load of a food based on the amount and type of minerals it contains.

The impact of acid-forming foods on PRAL is significant because consuming an excess of these foods can lead to an increased acid load in the body. This excess acid load may require the kidneys to work harder to maintain proper acid-base balance, potentially placing additional strain on their function.

Examples of Common Acid-Forming Foods

There are various types of acid-forming foods, and being aware of their acid-forming potential can help individuals make informed choices for their kidney health. Here are some common examples:

Meats: Animal proteins, such as beef, pork, lamb, and poultry, are considered acid-forming. These proteins contain sulfur-containing amino acids that, when metabolized, produce sulfuric acid as a byproduct.

Dairy Products: Most dairy products, including milk, cheese, yogurt, and ice cream, have an acidifying effect due to their protein content. While dairy products also provide essential nutrients like calcium, it's important to consume them in moderation and consider lower-acid alternatives when necessary.

Processed and Refined Grains: Highly processed grains like white bread, white rice, and pasta are typically acid-forming. These foods undergo extensive processing, which strips away fiber and important nutrients, leaving behind mostly simple carbohydrates that contribute to acidity.

Processed Meats: Deli meats, sausages, bacon, and other processed meat products are often high in sodium, nitrates, and other additives. These processed meats are acid-forming and can be detrimental to kidney health when consumed in excess.

Soft Drinks and Sweetened Beverages: Carbonated soft drinks, energy drinks, sweetened juices, and sports drinks are acidic due to their high sugar content. Regular consumption of these beverages can contribute to acidity in the body.

Sweets and Desserts: Foods high in added sugars, such as cakes, cookies, pastries, and candies, are acid-forming. These sugary treats not only contribute to acid load but also often lack essential nutrients.

Alcohol: Alcoholic beverages, such as beer, wine, and spirits, have an acidifying effect on the body. Alcohol can also dehydrate the body, putting additional stress on the kidneys.

The Potential Effects of High-Acid Diets on Kidney Health

Consuming a diet high in acid-forming foods and maintaining an elevated acid load over time may have implications for kidney health. The kidneys play a vital role in maintaining the body's acid-base balance by excreting excess acid through urine. However, prolonged exposure to high levels of acid can place a burden on the kidneys, potentially impacting their function and contributing to the development or progression of kidney disease.

High-acid diets have been associated with an increased risk of kidney stone formation. The excess acid load can alter urine pH and promote the crystallization of certain minerals, such as calcium oxalate or uric acid, increasing the likelihood of kidney stone formation.

Furthermore, high-acid diets may exacerbate existing kidney conditions, such as chronic kidney disease (CKD). The kidneys of individuals with CKD may have reduced capacity to eliminate excess acid, leading to further acid retention and potential complications. Elevated acid levels can contribute to inflammation, oxidative stress, and tissue damage in the kidneys, potentially accelerating the progression of kidney disease.

It is important to note that while acid-forming foods can contribute to the body's acid load, a healthy diet should still include a variety of nutrient-rich foods. The goal is not to eliminate acid-forming foods entirely but to strike a balance with alkaline-forming foods, such as fruits and vegetables, to promote overall acid-base equilibrium.

By being aware of the acid-forming potential of certain foods and striving for a balanced diet, individuals can make informed choices that support kidney health and overall well-being.

EXPLORING ALKALINE-FORMING FOODS AND THEIR IMPACT ON PRAL

Alkaline-forming foods are an important component of a kidney-friendly diet as they can help counterbalance the acidity in the body and promote a more balanced acid-base environment. By understanding the impact of alkaline-forming foods on the PRAL, you can optimize your dietary choices to support kidney health.

Examples of Common Alkaline-Forming Foods

Incorporating a variety of alkaline-forming foods into your diet can help maintain a more alkaline state in the body. Here are some additional examples of common alkaline-forming foods:

Cruciferous Vegetables: Cruciferous vegetables, such as broccoli, cauliflower, Brussels sprouts, and cabbage, are excellent alkaline-forming options. They are not only rich in alkaline minerals but also provide essential vitamins, fiber, and antioxidants.

Leafy Greens: Leafy greens like spinach, Swiss chard, arugula, and lettuce are highly alkaline-forming. They are packed with nutrients, including calcium, magnesium, and potassium, which contribute to maintaining an alkaline balance.

Cucumbers: Cucumbers have a high water content and are known for their alkalizing properties. They are refreshing and can be enjoyed as a snack or added to salads and sandwiches.

Bell Peppers: Bell peppers, whether green, red, or yellow, have an alkaline-forming effect. They are also rich in vitamins A and C, making them a nutritious addition to your meals.

Citrus Fruits: In addition to lemons and oranges, other citrus fruits like grapefruits and limes have alkaline properties. They provide a burst of flavor and are a great source of vitamin C.

Herbal Teas: Many herbal teas, such as chamomile, peppermint, and ginger tea, have an alkaline-forming effect. These teas not only contribute to hydration but also offer various health benefits.

Quinoa: Quinoa is a versatile grain that is considered alkaline-forming. It is a good source of plant-based protein, fiber, and essential minerals.

Sprouts: Sprouts, including alfalfa sprouts, broccoli sprouts, and bean sprouts, are alkaline-forming and can be added to salads, sandwiches, or stir-fries for added nutrition.

Watermelon: Watermelon is not only hydrating but also alkaline-forming. It is a delicious and refreshing fruit to enjoy during the warmer months.

How Alkaline-Forming Foods Help Balance Acid-Base Levels

Alkaline-forming foods play a vital role in balancing acid-base levels in the body. They contain alkaline minerals like potassium, magnesium, and calcium, which help neutralize excess acids and maintain a more alkaline environment.

By including a variety of alkaline-forming foods in your diet, you can support the body's natural buffering systems and reduce the burden on the kidneys. These foods help prevent the accumulation of acid residues in the body, which can contribute to kidney damage and other health issues.

Incorporating alkaline-forming foods can also enhance the overall nutrient density of your diet. They provide essential vitamins, minerals, antioxidants, and fiber, which are essential for overall health and well-being.

INTERPRETING PRAL VALUES

Understanding how to interpret PRAL values for different foods is crucial for making informed choices and optimizing your kidney-friendly diet. By identifying foods with a high or low PRAL, you can adjust your dietary intake to promote a more balanced acid-base environment and support kidney health.

How to Interpret PRAL Values

PRAL values indicate the potential acid load a particular food may have on the body. The values are measured in milliequivalents per 100 grams (mEq/100g) of food. A positive PRAL value indicates that the food is acid-forming, meaning it may contribute to acidity in the body. Conversely, a negative PRAL value indicates that the food is alkaline-forming, helping to neutralize excess acidity.

Identifying Foods with a High PRAL and Low PRAL

When interpreting PRAL values, it's important to identify foods with a high PRAL, as these may have a more significant acid-forming effect on the body. Examples of foods with a high PRAL include processed meats, cheese, refined grains, and carbonated beverages. These foods should be consumed in moderation or replaced with lower PRAL alternatives.

On the other hand, foods with a low PRAL are more alkaline-forming and can help balance acid-base levels in the body.

Examples of foods with a low PRAL include most fruits, vegetables, legumes, whole grains, nuts, and seeds. These foods are beneficial for a kidney-friendly diet and should be emphasized.

Tips for Incorporating Low PRAL Foods into a Kidney-Friendly Diet

Incorporating low PRAL foods into your kidney-friendly diet can help maintain a balanced acid-base environment and support kidney health. Here are some tips to help you incorporate low PRAL foods:

Prioritize fruits and vegetables: Fruits and vegetables, particularly those with negative PRAL values, are excellent choices. Aim to include a variety of colorful fruits and vegetables in your meals and snacks.

Choose whole grains: Opt for whole grains such as quinoa, brown rice, and whole wheat bread. These options tend to have lower PRAL values compared to refined grains.

Include plant-based protein sources: Legumes, such as beans, lentils, and chickpeas, provide protein while contributing to a lower PRAL. Consider incorporating these plant-based protein sources into your diet.

Emphasize nuts and seeds: Nuts and seeds, such as almonds, walnuts, flaxseeds, and chia seeds, offer a range of health benefits and tend to have lower PRAL values. Enjoy them as a snack or add them to meals.

Minimize processed and high-acid foods: Limit or avoid

processed meats, high-sodium snacks, sugary drinks, and refined grains as they tend to have higher PRAL values.

Utilizing a food tracking app like Cronometer (http://go.dadvicetv.com/app) can be helpful in tracking PRAL values and making informed dietary choices. The app allows you to input and monitor the PRAL values of various foods, making it easier to maintain a kidney-friendly diet. By tracking your PRAL intake, you can ensure you are incorporating a balance of acid-forming and alkaline-forming foods to support kidney health.

Remember, achieving a balanced acid-base environment involves the overall composition of your diet rather than focusing solely on individual foods. Aim for a diet that emphasizes whole, unprocessed foods, incorporates a variety of fruits and vegetables, and maintains a proper balance between acid-forming and alkaline-forming foods.

PRAL AND THE KIDNEY-FRIENDLY DIET

Understanding the role of PRAL in optimizing the kidney-friendly diet is essential for maintaining a balanced acid-base environment and supporting kidney health. By incorporating strategies to balance PRAL through food choices and incorporating PRAL awareness into meal planning and food selection, you can create a more kidney-friendly and health-promoting diet.

The Role of PRAL in Optimizing the Kidney-Friendly Diet

PRAL plays a significant role in the kidney-friendly diet as it helps assess the potential acid load that different foods may have on the body. By optimizing PRAL, you can create a diet that promotes a balanced acid-base environment, which is crucial for kidney health. A diet that is too acidic can put additional stress on the kidneys, potentially exacerbating kidney damage and impairing their function. Balancing PRAL helps reduce this burden and supports overall kidney health.

Strategies for Balancing PRAL through Food Choices

Achieving a balanced PRAL involves making strategic food choices to minimize the acid load on the body. Here are some strategies for balancing PRAL in your diet:

Emphasize alkaline-forming foods: Prioritize foods with a negative PRAL value, such as fruits, vegetables, legumes, and certain whole grains. These foods are alkaline-forming and can help neutralize excess acidity in the body.

Moderate acid-forming foods: While it's important to reduce the consumption of acid-forming foods, such as processed meats, cheese, and refined grains, you don't need to eliminate them entirely. Instead, aim to consume them in moderation and balance them with alkaline-forming foods.

Consider PRAL when meal planning: Incorporate PRAL awareness into your meal planning process. Aim to create meals that include a variety of low PRAL foods, such as salads with leafy greens, vegetable stir-fries, and plant-based protein sources like lentils or tofu.

Pay attention to cooking methods: Some cooking methods can impact the PRAL of foods.

- **Boiling**: Boiling is a cooking method that involves immersing food in boiling water. It is generally considered a neutral cooking method in terms of PRAL. Boiling can help remove some of the water-soluble minerals from food, including potassium, which may slightly reduce the acid load of the cooked food.

- **Steaming**: Steaming is a gentle cooking method that uses steam to cook food. Steaming helps retain the natural flavors, nutrients, and alkaline-forming properties of foods. It is considered a kidney-friendly cooking method as it does not add any additional acid load to the food.

- **Baking or Roasting**: Baking or roasting involves cooking food in dry heat in an oven. This cooking method can enhance the flavors and textures of food without significantly altering the acid-base balance. However, it's important to note that adding certain acidic ingredients or marinades to the food before baking or roasting can increase the overall acid load.

- **Grilling**: Grilling can add a smoky and charred flavor to food but may also contribute to the formation of advanced glycation end products (AGEs) that have been associated with inflammation and potential health risks. While grilling can be enjoyed in moderation, it's advisable to avoid excessive charring or burning of foods to minimize the formation of potentially harmful compounds.

- **Stir-Frying**: Stir-frying involves cooking food quickly in a small amount of oil over high heat. This cooking method helps retain the color, texture, and nutrients of the ingredients while minimizing the loss of water-soluble vitamins. Stir-frying is generally considered a kidney-friendly cooking method as it preserves the alkaline-forming properties of many vegetables and proteins.

Incorporating PRAL Awareness into Meal Planning and Food Selection

Incorporating PRAL awareness into your meal planning and food selection process can help you make more informed choices and create a kidney-friendly diet. Here are some tips to consider:

Read food labels: Pay attention to PRAL values when reading food labels. Look for products that have lower PRAL values or choose whole, unprocessed foods that are naturally lower in acidity.

Utilize resources and apps: Use resources and apps that provide PRAL information for different foods. Cronometer is one example of an app that allows you to track PRAL values, making it easier to monitor and adjust your dietary choices accordingly.

Seek guidance from a renal dietitian: Work with a renal dietitian who can provide personalized guidance on balancing PRAL in your diet. They can help you create meal plans, suggest suitable food swaps, and ensure your overall dietary approach supports kidney health.

By incorporating PRAL awareness into your meal planning and food selection, you can make more intentional choices to create a kidney-friendly diet that supports a balanced acid-base environment.

LIMITATIONS AND CONSIDERATIONS

While PRAL is a valuable tool in assessing the acid load of foods and its impact on kidney health, it's important to acknowledge its limitations and consider individual variations in acid-base balance and dietary needs. Here are some key considerations to keep in mind:

Limitations of PRAL as a Sole Measure

While PRAL provides valuable insights into the potential acid load of foods, it should not be the sole determinant of dietary choices. It's important to consider other factors such as overall nutrient composition, portion sizes, and the overall balance of the diet. PRAL values are based on laboratory analyses and may not fully reflect how different foods are metabolized and their impact on the body's acid-base balance. Therefore, it's crucial to interpret PRAL values in the context of an overall balanced and varied diet.

Individual Variations in Acid-Base Balance and Dietary Needs

It's essential to recognize that acid-base balance can vary among individuals based on factors such as genetics, overall health status, and specific kidney function. Some individuals may naturally have a more alkaline or acidic pH balance, and their dietary needs may differ. Additionally, other health conditions and medications may influence acid-base balance. Therefore, it's important to consider individual variations and work closely with a healthcare professional, such as a renal dietitian, to tailor dietary recommendations to your specific needs.

Furthermore, individual dietary needs go beyond acid-base balance. While PRAL focuses on acid-forming and alkaline-forming foods, it's important to consider other aspects of a kidney-friendly diet, such as managing sodium, phosphorus, potassium, and fluid intake. These factors play a significant role in kidney health and overall well-being. A comprehensive approach that considers multiple dietary factors is essential for optimizing kidney health and managing kidney disease effectively.

HEALTH FOOD SWAPS: NOURISHING YOUR KIDNEYS WITH DELICIOUS ALTERNATIVES

When faced with the challenge of adopting a kidney-friendly diet, it's natural to feel overwhelmed and concerned about finding suitable food options. The misconception that following a kidney-friendly diet means limited and tasteless meals can be discouraging. However, at Dadvice TV, we believe that nourishing your kidneys can also be a journey of exploring new flavors and discovering delicious alternatives. By incorporating simple food swaps into your routine, you can gradually transition to a healthier and more kidney-friendly way of eating without sacrificing taste or variety.

UNDERSTANDING THE DADVICE TV METHOD

The Dadvice TV method encourages finding healthier alternatives to replace common unhealthy foods. Rather than focusing on deprivation, this approach empowers you to make positive choices and enjoy a wide range of flavorful options. By swapping out ingredients or choosing kidney-friendly alternatives, you can create a satisfying and nutritious meal plan that supports your kidney health.

Snack Swaps:

Snacking is an essential part of our daily routine, but it's important to choose snacks that are low in sodium and kidney-friendly. Instead of reaching for high-sodium options like chips or processed snacks, consider these healthier alternatives:

- Fresh fruit slices with a sprinkle of cinnamon for a naturally sweet and refreshing snack.

- Homemade popcorn seasoned with herbs and spices instead of pre-packaged microwave popcorn.

- Roasted chickpeas or edamame as a crunchy and protein-rich option.

- Greek yogurt topped with berries and a drizzle of honey for a creamy and nutritious treat.

- Raw vegetable sticks such as carrots, celery, and bell peppers with a side of hummus for a satisfying crunch.

Meal Swaps:

Transforming your main meals into kidney-friendly options is easier than you think. Here are some flavorful swaps to consider:

- Swap out high-sodium condiments like soy sauce with low-sodium alternatives such as tamari or coconut aminos.

- Opt for lean proteins like skinless chicken, turkey, or fish instead of processed meats or fatty cuts of meat.

- Choose whole grains like quinoa, brown rice, or whole

wheat pasta instead of refined grains.

- Incorporate a variety of colorful vegetables into your meals, such as leafy greens, bell peppers, carrots, and broccoli, to boost the nutritional value.

- Experiment with different herbs and spices to enhance the flavor of your dishes without relying on excessive salt.

- Use olive oil or avocado oil instead of butter or margarine for healthier fats.

- Prepare homemade sauces and dressings using fresh ingredients and herbs to control sodium and sugar content.

Beverage Swaps:

Staying hydrated is crucial for kidney health, but it's important to be mindful of your beverage choices. Consider these kidney-friendly swaps:

- Replace sugary sodas and fruit juices with infused water by adding slices of cucumber, lemon, or fresh mint for a refreshing twist.

- Opt for herbal teas or unsweetened iced tea instead of sugary or caffeinated beverages.

- Enjoy a glass of low-fat milk or dairy alternatives like almond or oat milk as a source of calcium and vitamin D.

- Make your own fresh fruit smoothies with low-potassium options like berries and apples, using water or low-potassium milk as a base.

Dessert Swaps:

Indulging in a sweet treat can still be part of a kidney-friendly diet. Try these delicious dessert swaps:

- Choose fresh fruits or low-potassium options like

berries, apples, or pears instead of high-potassium fruits like bananas or oranges.

· Prepare homemade desserts using sugar substitutes like stevia or monk fruit sweeteners.

· Enjoy a small portion of sorbet or frozen yogurt instead of high-sugar ice creams.

· Make a refreshing fruit salad with a variety of fruits and a sprinkle of lime juice for added flavor.

Making simple food swaps is a practical and enjoyable way to embark on your kidney-friendly journey. By gradually incorporating healthier alternatives into your diet, you'll discover a world of delicious options that support your kidney health without compromising on taste. The Dadvice TV approach encourages you to explore, experiment, and find joy in nourishing your body while taking care of your kidneys. So, don't be afraid to start swapping and savoring the flavorful possibilities that await you on your path to a thriving life with kidney disease.

COOKING METHODS: UNLEASHING THE FLAVOR, PRESERVING KIDNEY HEALTH

Cooking methods can significantly impact the nutritional composition and overall healthiness of meals, especially for individuals with kidney disease. In this chapter, we will explore various cooking methods and their suitability for a kidney-friendly diet. By understanding which methods to embrace and which to avoid, you can unleash the flavor of your meals while preserving the health of your kidneys.

RECOMMENDED COOKING METHODS

Boiling: Boiling is a simple and effective cooking method that helps retain the nutrients in food without the need for added fats or oils. It is ideal for vegetables, grains, and legumes. By boiling foods, you can reduce their potassium and sodium content, making them more kidney-friendly. Popular foods for boiling include broccoli, carrots, quinoa, and lentils.

Steaming: Steaming is another excellent cooking method for kidney-friendly meals. It preserves the natural flavors, textures, and nutrients of food without the need for excessive fats or oils. Steaming is particularly suitable for vegetables, fish, and poultry. It helps retain moisture while minimizing potassium and sodium levels. Try steaming vegetables like asparagus, cauliflower, and Brussels sprouts for a nutrient-packed side dish.

Baking: Baking is a versatile method that allows you to cook a wide range of foods while minimizing the need for added fats. It is ideal for proteins like chicken, fish, and tofu, as well as for certain vegetables. Baking can enhance the flavors and textures of foods without compromising their nutritional value. Popular kidney-friendly options for baking include baked chicken breasts, roasted salmon, and baked sweet potatoes.

Grilling: Grilling adds a delightful smoky flavor to foods without the need for excessive fats or oils. It is a great option for lean meats, fish, and vegetables. Grilling helps drain excess fat from meats, making it a heart-healthy and kidney-friendly choice. Enjoy grilled chicken breasts, fish fillets, and skewered vegetables for a delicious and nutritious meal.

Stir-Frying (One of my personal favorite methods): Stir-frying is a fantastic cooking method that combines high heat with minimal oil. It involves quickly cooking bite-sized pieces of food in a hot pan or wok, allowing for maximum flavor and nutrient retention. Stir-frying is ideal for vegetables, lean proteins, and even tofu. It helps preserve the natural colors, textures, and flavors of ingredients while minimizing the need for excessive fats or oils. Try stir-frying colorful bell peppers, snap peas, and lean strips of chicken or shrimp for a vibrant and kidney-friendly stir-fry dish.

Air Frying: Air frying is a relatively new cooking method that uses hot air circulation to cook food, giving it a crispy texture without the need for excessive oil. It can be a great alternative to deep-frying, as it reduces fat intake while still providing a satisfying crunch. Air frying is suitable for items like french fries, chicken wings, and vegetable chips. For an amazing roasted potatoes alternative, try air frying radishes (special thanks to Jen Hernandez of Plant-Powered Kidneys for this delicious recommendation).

COOKING METHODS TO LIMIT OR AVOID

Frying: Frying involves submerging food in hot oil, which can increase its fat content and potentially introduce harmful substances. Fried foods are typically high in calories, unhealthy fats, and sodium, making them less suitable for a kidney-friendly diet. Limit your consumption of deep-fried foods like French fries, fried chicken, and battered snacks.

Braising: Braising involves searing meat in oil, then cooking it slowly in liquid. While this method can yield tender and flavorful results, it often requires higher amounts of added fats and may result in higher sodium content. Opt for alternative cooking methods to minimize fat and sodium intake.

By choosing the right cooking methods, you can transform ordinary ingredients into flavorful and kidney-friendly meals. Embrace boiling, steaming, baking, grilling, and stir-frying as preferred methods, as they retain nutrients, minimize added fats and oils, and reduce sodium and potassium levels. Stir-frying, in particular, offers a quick and delicious way to incorporate a variety of colorful vegetables and lean proteins into your diet. Limit or avoid frying and braising, as they can add excessive fats and sodium to your diet. Remember, variety is key, so experiment with different cooking methods to keep your meals exciting and enjoyable while prioritizing the health of your kidneys.

LEACHING POTASSIUM: A STRATEGY TO REDUCE POTASSIUM CONTENT IN FOODS

In managing chronic kidney disease or hyperkalemia (elevated potassium levels), your healthcare team may instruct you to reduce your potassium intake. One technique that can be employed is leaching, a process that involves soaking or boiling foods to remove some of their potassium content. In this chapter, we will delve into the concept of leaching potassium, discuss foods that can be leached, and provide detailed instructions on how to leach potassium from potatoes —a popular and versatile food.

UNDERSTANDING LEACHING POTASSIUM

Leaching is a culinary technique that helps decrease the potassium content of certain foods. Potassium is a mineral found naturally in many foods and is essential for various bodily functions. However, excessive potassium levels can be harmful to individuals with compromised kidney function. By using leaching, some of the potassium in foods can be removed, making them more suitable for individuals on low-potassium diets.

The amount of potassium that can be removed from food through leaching can vary depending on several factors, including the specific food item, the duration of soaking, and the temperature of the water used. While leaching can effectively reduce potassium levels, it is important to note that it may not completely eliminate potassium from the food.

Studies have shown that leaching techniques can remove a significant portion of potassium from certain foods. For example, research published in the Journal of Renal Nutrition has indicated that soaking potatoes in water for several hours or overnight can remove approximately 30% to 50% of the potassium content. Similarly, leaching legumes, such as beans or lentils, can result in potassium reduction by approximately 20% to 30%.

It is worth noting that the effectiveness of leaching may vary depending on the food item and its initial potassium content. Foods with higher potassium levels may still contain a substantial amount of potassium even after leaching. Therefore, it is crucial to work with a healthcare professional or renal dietitian who can provide personalized guidance on potassium restriction and appropriate leaching techniques based on individual needs and dietary requirements.

FOODS THAT CAN BE LEACHED

Several food items can undergo leaching to reduce their potassium content. These include:

Potatoes: Potatoes are a common staple in many diets and are known for their relatively high potassium content. Leaching can significantly reduce the potassium levels in potatoes, making them a viable option for individuals with potassium restrictions.

Vegetables: Certain vegetables, such as carrots, green beans, and winter squash, can also be leached to decrease their potassium content.

Fruits: Fruits like apples and pears can undergo leaching to reduce their potassium levels, particularly when used in cooking or baking.

Legumes: Legumes, such as beans and lentils, are nutritious sources of protein and fiber. Leaching can be employed to reduce their potassium content, making them more kidney-friendly.

Grains: Certain grains, including rice and oats, can be subjected to leaching to lower their potassium levels, providing options for individuals with dietary potassium restrictions.

LEACHING POTASSIUM FROM POTATOES

Potatoes are a versatile and widely consumed food, making them an excellent candidate for leaching. Here is a step-by-step guide on how to leach potassium from potatoes:

1. Peel and chop the potatoes: Start by peeling the potatoes to remove the skin. Then, chop them into small, uniform pieces. This will help facilitate the leaching process.

2. Rinse the potatoes: Place the chopped potatoes in

a colander and rinse them thoroughly under cold running water. This initial rinse helps remove any loose potassium on the surface.

3. Soak the potatoes: Transfer the rinsed potatoes to a large bowl and cover them with cold water. Allow them to soak for a minimum of two hours, but preferably overnight. The longer the soaking time, the more potassium will be leached out.

4. Drain and rinse again: After soaking, drain the water from the bowl and rinse the potatoes once more under cold running water. This final rinse helps remove any remaining potassium that has been released into the water.

5. Cooking the potatoes: Proceed to cook the leached potatoes according to your desired recipe. Boiling or steaming the potatoes is a common method for preparation. Remember to use fresh water for cooking to avoid reintroducing potassium.

THE BENEFITS OF LEACHING POTASSIUM

Leaching potassium from foods offers several benefits, especially for individuals with specific dietary requirements. Here are some key advantages:

Reduced Potassium Intake: Leaching allows individuals to enjoy a broader range of foods that are typically high in potassium while managing their potassium intake. This can help maintain optimal potassium levels and support overall health.

Increased Food Choices: By employing leaching techniques, individuals with potassium restrictions can expand their food choices and enjoy a more diverse and satisfying diet. This can promote adherence to dietary recommendations and improve overall dietary satisfaction.

Improved Nutritional Balance: Leaching helps balance the nutritional composition of foods by reducing their potassium content. This allows individuals to incorporate nutrient-rich ingredients, such as potatoes or legumes, into their meals without compromising their dietary restrictions.

SCIENTIFIC SUPPORT AND SOURCES

The effectiveness of leaching as a potassium reduction method has been examined in scientific studies. For example, a study published in the Journal of Renal Nutrition in 2016 investigated the effects of leaching on the potassium content of potatoes and other vegetables. The findings demonstrated that leaching significantly reduced the potassium levels in these foods, making them more suitable for individuals with kidney disease or hyperkalemia.

Another study published in the Journal of Renal Nutrition in 2012 explored the impact of different cooking methods, including leaching, on the potassium content of legumes. The results indicated that leaching effectively reduced potassium levels in legumes, supporting its use as a strategy for potassium reduction.

Leaching potassium is a practical and effective method for reducing the potassium content of certain foods. By employing leaching techniques, individuals with specific dietary restrictions, such as those with CKD or hyperkalemia, can expand their food choices and enjoy a more varied and balanced diet. However, it is important to note that the extent of potassium reduction may vary depending on factors such as soaking time, temperature, and the specific food being leached.

DINING OUT AND TRAVELING TIPS

Dining out and traveling can present unique challenges for individuals managing kidney disease. However, with proper planning and knowledge, it is possible to navigate these situations while making kidney-conscious choices. In this chapter, we will explore strategies and tips to help you stay on track with your kidney-friendly diet while enjoying meals at restaurants and traveling.

NAVIGATING RESTAURANT MENUS AND MAKING KIDNEY-CONSCIOUS CHOICES

When dining out, it's important to be mindful of your dietary needs and make kidney-conscious choices. By understanding how to navigate restaurant menus, you can make informed decisions that align with your kidney health goals. Here are some detailed tips to help you in this process:

Research and Plan Ahead:

Before visiting a restaurant, take the time to research their menu online, if available. Look for restaurants that offer healthier options or those that cater to specific dietary needs, such as low-sodium or kidney-friendly dishes. Reviewing the menu in advance allows you to identify suitable choices and plan your order accordingly.

Read Menu Descriptions Carefully:

When you're at the restaurant, pay close attention to the menu descriptions of the dishes. Look for keywords that may indicate higher sodium or phosphorus content, such as "smoked," "pickled," "brined," or "creamy." Opt for dishes that are described as "grilled," "baked," "steamed," or "fresh," as these are more likely to be lower in sodium and healthier overall.

Customize Your Order:

Don't hesitate to ask for modifications to suit your dietary requirements. Most restaurants are willing to accommodate special requests. For example, you can ask for sauces, dressings, or gravies to be served on the side so you can control the amount you consume. Requesting adjustments like reducing salt, omitting high-phosphorus ingredients, or substituting certain ingredients can help make the dish more kidney-friendly.

Choose Lean Protein Sources:

When selecting a protein source, opt for lean options such as skinless poultry, fish, or legumes. These choices are lower in saturated fat and phosphorus compared to fatty cuts of meat or processed meats. You can also request that your protein be prepared without added salt or seasonings high in sodium.

Be Mindful of Sodium Content:

Sodium can be a significant concern for individuals with kidney disease. Be aware of hidden sources of sodium in restaurant dishes, such as sauces, dressings, marinades, and seasoning blends. Ask for these to be served on the side so you can control the amount you consume. Alternatively, inquire about low-sodium alternatives or ask if dishes can be prepared without added salt.

Control Portion Sizes:

Restaurant portions are often larger than what is recommended for a kidney-friendly diet. Practice portion control by sharing a meal with a dining companion, requesting a half portion, or asking for a to-go container to save leftovers for another meal. This helps you manage your nutrient intake and prevent overeating.

Seek Out Healthier Cooking Methods:

Choose dishes that are prepared using healthier cooking methods such as grilling, baking, or steaming. These methods minimize the need for added fats and are generally lower in sodium compared to fried or heavily sauced options. Ask if substitutions can be made, such as steamed vegetables instead of fries or a grilled protein option instead of a breaded one.

Stay Mindful of Fluid Intake:

If you're managing fluid intake as part of your kidney health plan, be mindful of beverages when dining out. Opt for water or unsweetened beverages instead of sugary drinks or those high in sodium. Limiting alcohol and caffeine intake can also be beneficial for fluid management.

Remember, each restaurant and menu will offer different choices, so it's important to assess the options available and make the best decision based on your dietary needs. Don't hesitate to communicate with the server or chef about your dietary requirements and ask questions about the preparation of dishes. By being proactive and informed, you can make kidney-conscious choices while enjoying a dining experience outside of your home.

STRATEGIES FOR STAYING ON TRACK WHILE TRAVELING

Traveling can present unique challenges when it comes to maintaining a kidney-friendly diet. However, with careful planning and a proactive mindset, you can stay on track with your dietary goals even when away from home. Here are some detailed strategies to help you navigate your travels while prioritizing your kidney health:

Plan Ahead:

Before embarking on your trip, take the time to plan ahead for your meals. Research the destination's local cuisine and identify restaurants or grocery stores that offer kidney-friendly options. Look for eateries that prioritize fresh ingredients, lean proteins, and low-sodium preparations. Knowing where to find suitable meals or ingredients in advance can alleviate stress and make it easier to stick to your dietary requirements.

Pack Kidney-Friendly Snacks:

Bringing kidney-friendly snacks with you is a great way to ensure you have suitable options readily available, especially during long flights, road trips, or when access to suitable food is limited. Consider packing snacks such as low-sodium nuts, dried fruits, unsalted rice cakes, or homemade trail mix. These snacks can help you avoid unhealthy choices and keep your energy levels stable throughout your journey.

Research Local Food Options:

Take the opportunity to explore local food markets or specialty stores at your travel destination. These places often offer fresh produce, lean proteins, and kidney-friendly ingredients. Engage with locals and inquire about traditional dishes that align with your dietary needs. This allows you to enjoy the local cuisine while making mindful choices that support your kidney health.

Communicate Your Dietary Needs:

When dining out, don't hesitate to communicate your dietary needs to restaurant staff. Explain your restrictions and ask for modifications to suit your requirements. Most establishments are willing to accommodate special requests, such as reducing sodium or omitting certain ingredients. Clear communication ensures that your meals are prepared in a way that aligns with your dietary guidelines.

Pack Essential Medications and Supplies:

Ensure that you have an ample supply of your necessary medications and medical supplies for the duration of your trip. It's always advisable to bring extra medication in case of unexpected delays or emergencies. Pack your medications in your carry-on luggage to avoid any issues with lost or delayed checked baggage.

Stay Hydrated:

Maintaining proper hydration is crucial for kidney health, especially when traveling. Carry a refillable water bottle with you and drink fluids regularly throughout the day. Remember to adjust your fluid intake based on your individual needs and any fluid restrictions recommended by your healthcare team. If traveling to an area with limited access to safe drinking water, consider purchasing bottled water or using water purification methods.

Seek Out Local, Kidney-Friendly Options:

Explore local restaurants that offer healthier choices and cater to dietary restrictions. Seek out restaurants that emphasize fresh ingredients, grilled or baked preparations, and low-sodium seasonings. Local cuisine can be a delightful way to experience new flavors while ensuring you stay on track with your kidney-friendly diet.

Stay Mindful of Portion Sizes:

While traveling, it's common to encounter larger portion sizes at restaurants and food establishments. Be mindful of portion sizes and practice moderation. Consider sharing meals with travel companions or packing leftovers for later consumption. This helps you control your nutrient intake and prevent overeating.

Utilize Technology and Apps:

Take advantage of technology and smartphone apps that can assist you in making healthier choices while traveling. There are apps available that provide restaurant recommendations, highlight healthier menu options, or even help you locate grocery stores with kidney-friendly products. These tools can make it easier to stay on track and find suitable options wherever you are.

COMMUNICATION TIPS FOR SPECIAL DIETARY NEEDS

Effectively communicating your special dietary needs is crucial when dining out or traveling. By clearly expressing your requirements and advocating for yourself, you can ensure that your dietary needs are understood and accommodated. Here are some detailed communication tips to help you navigate situations where special dietary needs are involved:

Be Confident and Assertive:

When communicating your special dietary needs, it's important to be confident and assertive. Remember that your health is a priority, and you have the right to advocate for yourself. Approach conversations with restaurant staff or travel providers in a polite but firm manner, clearly expressing your dietary restrictions and requirements.

Plan Ahead and Research:

Before dining out or traveling, research and plan ahead to identify suitable options. Familiarize yourself with the local cuisine and learn about common ingredients and preparation methods. This knowledge will help you communicate your needs more effectively and make informed choices.

Clearly Explain Your Dietary Restrictions:

When discussing your dietary needs, clearly explain your restrictions and the reasons behind them. Whether it's low sodium, phosphorus, or specific dietary guidelines, provide a brief explanation of why these restrictions are essential for your health. This can help restaurant staff or travel providers understand the importance of meeting your needs.

Ask Questions:

Don't hesitate to ask questions about the menu, ingredients, or preparation methods. Inquire about specific dishes, cooking techniques, or the possibility of modifications. By asking questions, you can gather the necessary information to make informed decisions about your meals.

Use Specific Language:

Use specific language when describing your dietary restrictions. Instead of general statements like "I need to eat healthy" or "I have dietary restrictions," be specific about what you can and cannot consume. For example, you might say, "I need to avoid foods high in sodium due to kidney disease," or "I cannot consume dairy products because of lactose intolerance." Using clear and concise language helps avoid confusion and ensures your needs are accurately understood.

Carry a "Dietary Alert" Card:

Consider carrying a small card or note that outlines your specific dietary needs. This card can provide important details about your restrictions, such as low-sodium or low-phosphorus requirements, and can be presented to restaurant staff or travel providers. Including your name, contact information, and any emergency instructions can be helpful as well.

Utilize Translation Tools:

If traveling to a country where the primary language is different from your own, consider utilizing translation tools or smartphone apps. These tools can help bridge the communication gap by translating key phrases or dietary restrictions. Preparing translations in advance can facilitate effective communication and ensure your needs are understood.

Express Gratitude and Appreciation:

When your dietary needs are accommodated, express gratitude and appreciation to the restaurant staff or travel providers. A simple thank you can go a long way in acknowledging their efforts to meet your requirements. This positive interaction fosters understanding and encourages future support.

KIDNEY-FRIENDLY EXAMPLES FROM POPULAR RESTAURANTS

While specific menu items may vary by location, here are some recommendations from popular restaurant chains that can serve **as a starting point** for making healthier choices. Note – dining out is generally not kidney-friendly and should be considered an occasional treat and not the primary source of your meals:

Subway:

- Choose a 6-inch or footlong sandwich on whole grain bread with lean protein options like turkey, chicken breast, or roast beef.

- Load up on a variety of fresh vegetables, such as lettuce, tomatoes, cucumbers, and bell peppers.

- Opt for low-sodium or vinegar-based dressings and avoid high-sodium condiments like mayonnaise or pickles.

Chipotle:

- Opt for a salad bowl or burrito bowl as the base instead of a burrito or tacos.

- Choose lean protein options like chicken or steak and ask for smaller portions.

- Load up on kidney-friendly toppings like black beans, fajita vegetables, salsa, guacamole, and lettuce.

- Be mindful of sodium content and avoid adding extra cheese, sour cream, or high-sodium sauces.

Olive Garden:

- Choose grilled or broiled seafood options like salmon or shrimp as your protein.

- Opt for pasta dishes with tomato-based sauces instead of creamy sauces.

- Request for a side of steamed vegetables or a side salad with low-sodium dressing.

- Be mindful of portion sizes and consider splitting a meal or taking leftovers for later.

Panera Bread:

- Select soups with kidney-friendly options like vegetable-based or broth-based soups.

- Opt for salads with lean protein sources like grilled chicken or shrimp.

- Choose whole grain bread options for sandwiches and opt for low-sodium or oil-based dressings.

- Avoid high-sodium deli meats, creamy sauces, and added cheeses.

Outback Steakhouse:

- Choose lean cuts of grilled or roasted steak, such as sirloin or filet.

- Opt for plain baked potatoes or steamed vegetables as side dishes.

- Request for sauces, dressings, or gravies to be served on the side to control sodium intake.

- Be mindful of portion sizes and consider sharing a meal or saving leftovers for later.

McDonald's:

- Choose grilled chicken options like the Grilled Chicken Sandwich or Grilled Chicken Salad.

- Opt for side salads with low-sodium dressings or a fruit cup as a healthier side option.

- Request for no added salt or seasoning on your food.

- Avoid high-sodium sauces, crispy chicken options, and heavily salted sides.

Wendy's:

- Choose the Grilled Chicken Sandwich or Grilled Chicken Wrap as healthier protein options.
- Opt for side salads with low-sodium dressings or apple slices instead of fries.
- Be mindful of sodium content and choose items without excessive sauces or condiments.
- Avoid breaded or fried items and high-sodium toppings like bacon or cheese.

Taco Bell:

- Opt for protein options like grilled chicken or steak in tacos, bowls, or salads.
- Choose fresco-style options, which replace cheese and sauces with pico de gallo.
- Be mindful of sodium content and avoid high-sodium toppings like sour cream or guacamole.
- Consider ordering a side of black beans or seasoned rice as a kidney-friendly addition.

Applebee's:

- Choose grilled or broiled protein options like chicken, shrimp, or fish.
- Opt for steamed vegetables or side salads as healthy sides.
- Request for sauces, dressings, or gravies to be served on the side to control sodium intake.
- Be mindful of portion sizes and consider sharing a meal or taking leftovers for later.

Chili's:

- Choose grilled or roasted protein options like chicken,

salmon, or shrimp.

- Opt for steamed vegetables or side salads with low-sodium dressings as healthier sides.

- Request for sauces or dressings to be served on the side to control sodium intake.

- Avoid high-sodium toppings like bacon or crispy onions.

Chick-fil-A:

- Opt for grilled chicken options like the Grilled Chicken Sandwich or Grilled Chicken Cool Wrap.

- Choose side options like fruit cups or side salads instead of fries.

- Request for sauces to be served on the side to control sodium intake.

- Avoid breaded or fried items and high-sodium sauces like the Chick-fil-A Sauce.

Pizza Hut:

- Opt for thin crust pizzas with vegetable toppings and lean protein options like grilled chicken.

- Request for reduced sodium cheese or less cheese on your pizza.

- Be mindful of portion sizes and limit the number of slices consumed.

- Avoid high-sodium toppings like bacon or sausage.

Starbucks:

- Choose brewed coffee, unsweetened tea, or sugar-free beverages.

- Opt for plain oatmeal with added nuts or fresh fruits for a kidney-friendly breakfast option.

- Request for low-sodium options or ask for no added salt on sandwiches or wraps.

- Avoid high-sodium syrups, sauces, and sweetened beverages.

Red Lobster:

- Choose grilled or broiled seafood options like salmon, shrimp, or whitefish.
- Opt for steamed vegetables or side salads with low-sodium dressings as healthier sides.
- Request for sauces or dressings to be served on the side to control sodium intake.
- Be mindful of portion sizes and consider sharing a seafood platter or taking leftovers for later.

Denny's:

- Opt for egg-white omelets with vegetables or grilled chicken as a healthier protein option.
- Choose side options like fresh fruit or steamed vegetables.
- Request for no added salt or seasoning on your food.
- Avoid high-sodium items like bacon, sausages, or heavily salted side dishes.

Panda Express:

- Choose grilled or steamed protein options like grilled chicken or shrimp.
- Opt for vegetable-based dishes like steamed mixed vegetables or mixed greens.
- Be mindful of sodium content and limit or avoid high-sodium sauces like soy sauce or teriyaki sauce.
- Request for sauces to be served on the side to control sodium intake.

Olive Garden:

- Choose grilled or broiled seafood options like salmon or

shrimp as your protein.

- Opt for pasta dishes with tomato-based sauces instead of creamy sauces.

- Request for a side of steamed vegetables or a side salad with low-sodium dressing.

- Be mindful of portion sizes and consider splitting a meal or taking leftovers for later.

Papa John's:

- Opt for thin crust pizzas with vegetable toppings and lean protein options like grilled chicken.

- Request for reduced sodium cheese or less cheese on your pizza.

- Be mindful of portion sizes and limit the number of slices consumed.

- Avoid high-sodium toppings like bacon or sausage.

IHOP:

- Choose egg-white omelets with vegetables or lean protein options like grilled chicken or turkey bacon.

- Opt for side options like fresh fruit or steamed vegetables.

- Request for no added salt or seasoning on your food.

- Avoid high-sodium items like sausages, heavily salted pancakes, or syrup.

Burger King:

- Opt for grilled chicken sandwiches or burgers without cheese or mayonnaise.

- Choose side options like apple slices or side salads instead of fries.

- Be mindful of sodium content and avoid high-sodium condiments like ketchup or barbecue sauce.

- Request for no added salt or seasoning on your food.

Arby's:

- Choose lean protein options like roast turkey or roast chicken sandwiches.
- Opt for side options like side salads or apple slices instead of fries.
- Be mindful of sodium content and choose items without excessive sauces or condiments.
- Request for no added salt or seasoning on your food.

Jimmy John's:

- Choose sandwich options with lean proteins like turkey breast or roast beef.
- Opt for lettuce wraps or unwiches to reduce carbohydrate intake.
- Load up on fresh vegetables and choose lower-sodium condiments like mustard or vinegar.
- Be mindful of sodium content and avoid high-sodium deli meats or spreads.

Red Robin:

- Choose grilled chicken or turkey burgers as healthier protein options.
- Opt for whole wheat or lettuce wraps instead of regular buns.
- Load up on fresh toppings like lettuce, tomatoes, onions, and pickles.
- Request for no added salt or seasoning on your food and avoid high-sodium sauces or toppings.

Texas Roadhouse:

- Choose grilled or roasted protein options like grilled chicken or steak.

- Opt for plain baked potatoes or steamed vegetables as side dishes.

- Request for sauces or dressings to be served on the side to control sodium intake.

- Be mindful of portion sizes and consider sharing a meal or saving leftovers for later.

Del Taco:

- Choose grilled chicken or grilled shrimp options in tacos, burritos, or bowls.

- Opt for fresco-style options, which replace cheese and sauces with pico de gallo.

- Be mindful of sodium content and avoid high-sodium toppings like sour cream or guacamole.

- Consider ordering a side of black beans or seasoned rice as a kidney-friendly addition.

Outback Steakhouse:

- Choose grilled or roasted protein options like chicken, salmon, or shrimp.

- Opt for plain baked potatoes or steamed vegetables as side dishes.

- Request for sauces or dressings to be served on the side to control sodium intake.

- Be mindful of portion sizes and consider sharing a meal or saving leftovers for later.

Domino's:

- Choose thin crust pizzas with vegetable toppings and lean protein options like grilled chicken.

- Request for reduced sodium cheese or less cheese on your pizza.

- Be mindful of portion sizes and limit the number of slices consumed.

- Avoid high-sodium toppings like bacon or sausage.

Dairy Queen:

- Choose grilled chicken sandwiches or wraps without cheese or high-sodium sauces.

- Opt for side options like apple slices or a side salad instead of fries.

- Be mindful of sodium content and avoid high-sodium toppings like bacon or sauces.

- Request for no added salt or seasoning on your food.

Firehouse Subs:

- Opt for the "Under 500 Calories" menu options, which include a variety of lower-calorie and lower-sodium subs.

- Choose lean protein options like turkey or roast beef with plenty of fresh vegetables.

- Request for no added salt or seasoning on your sub.

- Be mindful of portion sizes and consider choosing a smaller size or saving half for later.

Jersey Mike's:

- Choose the "Sub in a Tub" option, which replaces the bread with a bed of lettuce for a low-carb and lower-sodium choice.

- Opt for lean protein options like turkey breast or grilled chicken.

- Load up on fresh vegetables and choose lower-sodium dressings or oil and vinegar.

- Be mindful of sodium content and avoid high-sodium toppings or condiments.

Boston Market:

- Choose roasted turkey breast or roasted chicken as

healthier protein options.

- Opt for steamed vegetables or side salads as healthy sides.
- Request for sauces or gravies to be served on the side to control sodium intake.
- Be mindful of portion sizes and consider sharing a meal or taking leftovers for later.

Five Guys:

- Choose the bunless option and have your burger wrapped in lettuce.
- Opt for single patty burgers and limit high-sodium toppings like bacon or cheese.
- Load up on fresh vegetable toppings like lettuce, tomatoes, onions, and pickles.
- Be mindful of sodium content and avoid excessive condiments or salted fries.

Sonic:

- Choose grilled chicken options like the Grilled Chicken Sandwich or Grilled Chicken Wrap.
- Opt for side options like apple slices or side salads instead of fries.
- Be mindful of sodium content and avoid high-sodium condiments like ketchup or barbecue sauce.
- Request for no added salt or seasoning on your food.

O'Charley's:

- Choose grilled or broiled protein options like chicken, salmon, or shrimp.
- Opt for steamed vegetables or side salads with low-sodium dressings as healthier sides.
- Request for sauces or dressings to be served on the side to control sodium intake.

- Be mindful of portion sizes and consider sharing a meal or taking leftovers for later.

P.F. Chang's:

- Choose steamed protein options like chicken, shrimp, or tofu.

- Opt for vegetable-based dishes like Buddha's Feast or Stir-Fried Eggplant.

- Be mindful of sodium content and avoid high-sodium sauces like soy sauce or hoisin sauce.

- Request for sauces to be served on the side to control sodium intake.

Buffalo Wild Wings:

- Opt for grilled chicken or unbreaded boneless wings as protein options.

- Choose sauces or seasonings with lower sodium content or request for sauces to be served on the side.

- Be mindful of portion sizes and limit the consumption of high-sodium sides like fries or cheese dips.

- Enjoy celery sticks as a low-sodium alternative for dipping.

BJ's Restaurant & Brewhouse:

- Choose grilled or roasted protein options like chicken, salmon, or steak.

- Opt for steamed vegetables or side salads with low-sodium dressings as healthier sides.

- Request for sauces or dressings to be served on the side to control sodium intake.

- Be mindful of portion sizes and consider sharing a meal or taking leftovers for later.

Yard House:

- Choose grilled or roasted protein options like chicken, salmon, or steak.
- Opt for side options like steamed vegetables or a side salad with low-sodium dressings.
- Request for sauces or dressings to be served on the side to control sodium intake.
- Be mindful of portion sizes and consider sharing a meal or taking leftovers for later.

Bahama Breeze Island Grille:

- Choose grilled seafood options like grilled salmon or shrimp.
- Opt for side options like steamed vegetables or a side salad with low-sodium dressings.
- Request for sauces or dressings to be served on the side to control sodium intake.
- Be mindful of portion sizes and consider sharing a meal or taking leftovers for later.

Maggiano's Little Italy:

- Choose grilled or roasted protein options like chicken, salmon, or steak.
- Opt for tomato-based pasta sauces instead of cream-based sauces.
- Request for sauces or dressings to be served on the side to control sodium intake.
- Be mindful of portion sizes and consider sharing a meal or taking leftovers for later.

The Cheesecake Factory:

- Choose grilled or roasted protein options like chicken, salmon, or steak.
- Opt for vegetable-based dishes like salads or roasted

vegetable plates.

- Request for sauces or dressings to be served on the side to control sodium intake.

- Be mindful of portion sizes and consider sharing a meal or taking leftovers for later.

Remember that while dining out can be accommodated to be kidney-friendly, it's important to view it as an **occasional activity** rather than a primary source for the majority of meals. With careful planning and communication, you can enjoy a kidney-friendly dining experience. However, keep in mind that the best approach to managing your kidney health is to prioritize home-cooked meals using fresh, kidney-friendly ingredients. This allows for better control over the nutritional content of your meals, ensuring they align with your dietary needs. Dining out should be seen as a special treat or a social occasion, while the majority of your meals are prepared at home, providing you with the best opportunity to maintain a kidney-friendly diet.

EXPLORING MINDFUL EATING FOR KIDNEY HEALTH

In today's fast-paced world, where distractions abound and meals are often rushed, the concept of mindful eating offers a refreshing approach to nourishing our bodies and supporting kidney health. Mindful eating is an ancient practice that invites us to engage with food in a more conscious and intentional way. It encourages us to slow down, savor each bite, and develop a deeper connection with the nourishment we provide our bodies.

At its core, mindful eating is about being fully present in the moment and paying attention to the entire eating experience – from selecting the ingredients and preparing the meal to savoring the flavors and listening to our body's signals of hunger and satiety. It involves bringing awareness to the thoughts, emotions, and sensations that arise as we eat, fostering a greater understanding of our relationship with food.

By incorporating mindful eating into our lives, we can transform our mealtimes into opportunities for self-care, self-awareness, and nurturing our bodies. This chapter will guide you through the principles and strategies of mindful eating, empowering you to develop a healthy relationship with food while supporting your kidney health.

THE IMPORTANCE OF MINDFUL EATING IN KIDNEY HEALTH

Mindful eating plays a pivotal role in supporting kidney health and overall well-being. By practicing mindful eating, we bring conscious awareness to our food choices, eating habits, and the impact they have on our kidneys. Here are several key reasons why mindful eating is of utmost importance for kidney health:

Portion Control: Mindful eating helps us tune in to our body's cues of hunger and fullness. By paying attention to these signals, we can better control our portion sizes, preventing overeating and reducing unnecessary strain on our kidneys. Portion control is especially crucial for individuals with kidney disease, as excess food intake can contribute to fluid retention, electrolyte imbalances, and overall kidney burden.

Optimal Nutrient Intake: Mindful eating allows us to make informed choices about the types of foods we consume, ensuring that we provide our bodies with the necessary nutrients for kidney health. By focusing on nutrient-dense whole foods, we can prioritize foods that support kidney function, such as those low in sodium, phosphorus, and potassium, while rich in essential vitamins, minerals, and antioxidants.

Blood Pressure Management: Mindful eating can help manage blood pressure, a critical aspect of kidney health. By being mindful of our sodium intake and choosing low-sodium options, we can reduce the risk of hypertension, a leading cause of kidney damage. Mindful eating also encourages us to incorporate foods that promote cardiovascular health, such as those rich in omega-3 fatty acids, which can help maintain healthy blood pressure levels.

Digestive Wellness: Mindful eating promotes healthy digestion, which is vital for optimal kidney health. By savoring each bite and chewing food thoroughly, we aid the digestive process, allowing our bodies to absorb nutrients more effectively. Mindful eating also reduces the likelihood of overeating, which can lead to indigestion, discomfort, and potential gastrointestinal issues that can impact kidney health.

Emotional Well-being: Mindful eating addresses the emotional aspect of our relationship with food. It encourages us to become more aware of emotional triggers, such as stress or boredom, that may influence our eating habits. By mindfully identifying and addressing these triggers, we can develop healthier coping mechanisms that don't involve emotional overeating or the consumption of foods that may negatively impact our kidney health.

Mind-Body Connection: Mindful eating fosters a deeper mind-body connection, allowing us to appreciate the connection between our food choices and how we feel physically and emotionally. By attuning ourselves to the nourishment we provide our bodies, we become more mindful of the impact our choices have on our overall well-being, including kidney health. This awareness empowers us to make conscious decisions that align with our health goals.

STRATEGIES FOR PRACTICING MINDFUL EATING AND ENJOYING MEALS

Create a Calm Eating Environment: Set aside dedicated time and space for your meals, free from distractions. Remove electronic devices, turn off the TV, and find a quiet area where you can focus on your food and the act of eating. Creating a calm environment allows you to fully engage your senses and be present with your meal.

Engage Your Senses: Before taking your first bite, take a moment to observe your meal with all your senses. Notice the colors, textures, and aromas of the food on your plate. Allow yourself to appreciate the visual appeal and enticing smells of your meal, building anticipation and excitement for the eating experience.

Slow Down and Chew Thoroughly: Practice eating at a slower pace and chew each bite thoroughly. Eating slowly gives your body time to register fullness and satiety cues, preventing overeating. Take the time to savor the flavors and textures of your food, fully experiencing the taste sensations as you chew.

Practice Mindful Portion Control: Be mindful of portion sizes and serve yourself appropriate amounts of food. Use smaller plates or bowls to create the illusion of a fuller plate. Take note of your body's hunger and fullness signals, stopping when you feel comfortably satisfied. Avoid the temptation to finish everything on your plate if you are already full.

Focus on Each Bite: Direct your attention to the present moment by focusing on each bite of food. Notice the flavors, textures, and the way the food feels in your mouth. Avoid rushing through your meal and instead appreciate the sensory experience of eating.

Cultivate Gratitude: Express gratitude for the nourishment provided by your meal. Reflect on the effort and care that went into preparing the food, from the farmers who grew it to the hands that cooked it. Take a moment to appreciate the journey of the food from farm to table, fostering a sense of gratitude for the sustenance it provides.

Practice Mindful Drinking: Extend the principles of mindful eating to your beverage consumption. Be aware of the sensations and flavors of the beverages you consume, such as water, herbal teas, or other kidney-friendly drinks. Sip slowly and enjoy the refreshment they offer.

Tune into Hunger and Fullness Cues: Develop a heightened awareness of your body's hunger and fullness cues. Before reaching for a snack or second helping, take a moment to assess if you are truly hungry or if you are eating out of habit, boredom, or emotions. Likewise, listen to your body when it signals that you are comfortably full and stop eating.

Practice Gratitude and Mindful Reflection: After you finish your meal, take a moment to express gratitude for the nourishment you received. Reflect on the experience of eating mindfully, noticing any thoughts or emotions that arise. Use this time to cultivate a sense of appreciation for the positive impact that mindful eating can have on your overall well-being.

BUILDING A POSITIVE RELATIONSHIP WITH FOOD AND PROMOTING WELL-BEING

Developing a positive relationship with food is an essential aspect of promoting overall well-being and supporting kidney health. It involves cultivating a balanced and mindful approach to nourishing our bodies while fostering a healthy mindset around food. Here are key strategies for building a positive relationship with food:

Embrace Food as Nourishment: Shift your perspective to view food as a source of nourishment, providing the essential nutrients your body needs to thrive. Recognize that every meal is an opportunity to nourish your body and support your kidney health. Appreciate the role that wholesome, nutrient-dense foods play in providing energy, supporting organ function, and maintaining overall well-being.

Practice Self-Compassion: Be kind to yourself and practice self-compassion in your relationship with food. Understand that healthy eating is a journey, and occasional deviations or indulgences are a normal part of life. Avoid guilt or judgment around food choices and instead focus on making balanced choices that support your overall health. Treat yourself with kindness and forgive yourself if you occasionally veer from your kidney-friendly diet.

Listen to Your Body: Cultivate awareness of your body's signals of hunger, fullness, and satisfaction. Learn to differentiate between physical hunger and emotional cues for eating. Honor your body's cues by eating when you're hungry and stopping when you're comfortably satisfied. Trust your body's wisdom and give yourself permission to enjoy food without restrictions or guilt.

Practice Mindful Awareness: Develop mindful awareness of your thoughts, emotions, and behaviors around food. Notice any patterns of emotional eating, stress-induced eating, or mindless snacking. Take time to reflect on the triggers that may influence your relationship with food and find healthier ways to address those emotions or stressors. Mindful awareness allows you to make conscious choices and respond to your body's true needs.

Foster a Balanced Approach: Strive for balance in your eating habits, incorporating a variety of nutrient-dense foods while allowing for occasional indulgences. Emphasize the importance of whole foods, such as fruits, vegetables, whole grains, lean proteins, and healthy fats, in your daily meals. Aim to create well-rounded, satisfying meals that provide a range of flavors, textures, and nutrients.

Practice Mindful Preparation: Engage in mindful preparation of your meals by participating in the cooking process. Choose fresh, high-quality ingredients and take pleasure in the act of preparing and cooking your meals. This involvement cultivates a deeper appreciation for the food you consume and strengthens your connection to the nourishment it provides.

Seek Support and Community: Surround yourself with a supportive community that shares similar health goals. Connect with others who are on a kidney health journey, whether through support groups, online communities, or local organizations. Sharing experiences, insights, and resources can provide encouragement, motivation, and a sense of belonging on your path to building a positive relationship with food.

Seek Professional Guidance: Consider working with a registered dietitian specializing in renal nutrition to receive personalized guidance and support. A renal dietitian can provide expert advice on meal planning, portion control, and incorporating kidney-friendly foods into your diet. They can also help address specific dietary restrictions or concerns, ensuring that your nutritional needs are met while promoting a positive relationship with food.

Maintaining a kidney-friendly diet can be a challenging endeavor, and it's important to approach it with flexibility and self-compassion. There may be times when you deviate from your planned diet due to various reasons or circumstances. In such instances, it is crucial to practice forgiveness and avoid being too hard on yourself. Here are key reasons why forgiving yourself is essential:

Recognize Your Humanity: It is important to acknowledge that we are all human and that deviations from our diet can occur from time to time. Life is full of unexpected events, celebrations, and social gatherings where adhering strictly to your kidney-friendly diet may not always be possible. It's normal to have moments of indulgence or veer off course, and forgiving yourself is a way to honor your humanity and avoid unnecessary self-judgment.

Avoid the Guilt and Shame Cycle: Dwelling in guilt and shame can create a negative cycle that impacts your overall well-being. When you feel guilty about not adhering to your diet, it can lead to negative self-talk and self-criticism, which can further perpetuate unhealthy behaviors or emotional eating. Forgiving yourself breaks this cycle, allowing you to move forward with a more positive mindset and a renewed commitment to your kidney health.

Embrace the Big Picture: While adhering to a kidney-friendly diet is important for managing kidney disease, it's crucial to keep in mind the bigger picture of your overall health and well-being. Focusing solely on occasional dietary lapses may cause undue stress and anxiety, which can be counterproductive to your overall health goals. Forgiving yourself allows you to adopt a more holistic perspective and recognize that your well-being is influenced by various factors beyond just diet.

Learn from the Experience: Instead of dwelling on the slip-up, use it as an opportunity for growth and learning. Reflect on what led to the deviation from your diet, whether it was an emotional trigger, a social event, or a moment of weakness. Understand the circumstances that contributed to the lapse and consider how you can better navigate similar situations in the future. By learning from the experience, you can develop strategies to prevent or minimize future deviations.

Reestablish Your Commitment: Forgiving yourself enables you to reestablish your commitment to your kidney health goals. Recognize that occasional lapses do not define your overall progress. Refocus on your motivation and remind yourself of the importance of following a kidney-friendly diet. Use the experience as a reminder of your commitment and find renewed determination to make positive choices moving forward.

Seek Support: Reach out to your support network, whether it be your healthcare team, family, or friends, and share your challenges and setbacks. Their understanding and encouragement can help you regain perspective and provide valuable support during moments of difficulty. Having someone to talk to, share experiences with, and seek guidance from can make the journey towards maintaining a kidney-friendly diet easier and more manageable.

Remember, forgiving yourself for occasional lapses is an act of self-compassion and a recognition of your journey's ups and downs. Embrace forgiveness as an opportunity for growth, learning, and renewed commitment to your kidney health. By approaching your dietary choices with self-compassion and understanding, you create a positive and sustainable mindset that supports your overall well-being.

BEYOND THE PLATE: LIFESTYLE AND WELLNESS

When it comes to supporting kidney health, incorporating complementary practices alongside a kidney-friendly diet can enhance your overall well-being and promote optimal kidney function. Consider the following practices:

Mind-Body Techniques: Mind-body techniques have been shown to reduce stress, promote relaxation, and improve overall well-being. These practices can include:

- **Meditation**: Engage in meditation, which involves focusing your attention and eliminating the stream of thoughts, promoting a sense of calm and relaxation. Regular meditation practice can help reduce stress, lower blood pressure, and improve mental clarity.

- **Deep Breathing Exercises**: Practice deep breathing exercises, such as diaphragmatic breathing or box breathing. These techniques involve taking slow, deep breaths, filling your abdomen with air, and exhaling fully. Deep breathing promotes relaxation, reduces anxiety, and helps manage stress.

- **Mindfulness**: Cultivate mindfulness by paying attention to the present moment without judgment. Mindfulness practices can include mindful eating, mindful walking, or mindful body scans. By being fully present, you can enhance your connection to your body, reduce stress, and improve overall well-being.

Yoga or Tai Chi: Incorporating gentle forms of exercise such as yoga or Tai Chi can provide numerous benefits for kidney health. These practices combine movement, breath control, and mindfulness to promote physical strength, flexibility, balance, and mental well-being. They also help reduce stress and support overall kidney health.

- Yoga: Explore yoga postures (asanas) and gentle stretches that can improve flexibility, muscle strength, and circulation. Yoga also emphasizes deep breathing, relaxation, and mindfulness, which can help manage stress and enhance kidney health.

- Tai Chi: Consider Tai Chi, a Chinese martial art that involves slow, flowing movements and deep breathing. Tai Chi promotes relaxation, balance, flexibility, and mental clarity. Regular practice can improve overall well-being and support kidney health.

Acupuncture: Acupuncture is an ancient practice that involves the insertion of thin needles into specific points of the body. This practice is believed to promote balance, stimulate healing, and support kidney health. Acupuncture may assist in managing symptoms related to kidney disease, such as pain, fatigue, sleep disturbances, and overall well-being. Consult with a qualified acupuncturist experienced in working with individuals with kidney disease.

Massage Therapy: Massage therapy offers a range of techniques that can promote relaxation, reduce muscle tension, improve circulation, and support overall well-being. Consider incorporating massage therapy into your self-care routine to help manage stress, improve lymphatic flow, and enhance kidney function. It's essential to choose a licensed massage therapist who is knowledgeable about working with individuals with kidney disease.

By embracing these complementary practices, you can enhance your kidney health and overall well-being. Explore different techniques, find what resonates with you, and integrate them into your daily life. Remember to consult with your healthcare team before beginning any new practices, especially if you have specific health concerns or conditions.

EXERCISE, STRESS MANAGEMENT, AND SLEEP FOR OPTIMAL WELL-BEING

When it comes to promoting optimal well-being and supporting kidney health, exercise, stress management, and quality sleep play vital roles. Here's a look at each of these components:

Exercise:

- Regular physical activity offers numerous benefits for both physical and mental health. Engaging in exercise can:

- Improve Cardiovascular Health: Cardiovascular exercises like brisk walking, cycling, swimming, or dancing help strengthen the heart and improve blood circulation. This promotes overall cardiovascular health, including kidney health.

- Maintain a Healthy Weight: Regular exercise aids in weight management, which is important for reducing the risk of chronic conditions such as obesity, diabetes, and high blood pressure. Maintaining a healthy weight is beneficial for kidney health as it helps prevent excessive stress on the kidneys.

- Support Kidney Function: Exercise promotes overall blood flow and oxygenation, which can support kidney function. It also helps maintain healthy blood pressure levels, reducing the risk of kidney damage. Consult with your healthcare professional to determine appropriate exercise intensity and duration based on your individual needs and health condition.

Stress Management:

- Chronic stress can negatively impact kidney health and overall well-being. Implementing effective stress management techniques can help:

- Reduce Stress Hormones: Engaging in stress-reducing activities like deep breathing exercises, meditation, or yoga can help lower the levels of stress hormones in your body. This promotes a sense of calm, relaxation, and mental well-being.

- Enhance Coping Mechanisms: Stress management techniques equip you with healthy coping strategies to navigate challenges and reduce the negative impact of stress on your overall health. Find activities that help you unwind, such as engaging in hobbies, spending time in nature, or listening to soothing music.

· Support Emotional Well-being: Prioritize self-care activities that nurture your emotional well-being. This may include journaling, practicing gratitude, spending quality time with loved ones, or seeking professional support when needed. Building emotional resilience can positively impact your ability to manage stress and promote overall well-being.

Sleep:

· Quality sleep is essential for your body's restorative processes and overall well-being. Consider the following to support restful sleep:

· Establish a Consistent Sleep Routine: Create a regular sleep schedule by going to bed and waking up at consistent times. This helps regulate your body's internal clock and promotes better sleep quality.

· Create a Sleep-Friendly Environment: Design your sleep environment to promote relaxation and restfulness. Ensure your bedroom is cool, quiet, and dark. Consider using comfortable bedding, earplugs, eye masks, or white noise machines if needed.

· Practice Relaxation Techniques: Incorporate relaxation techniques, such as deep breathing exercises or meditation, into your bedtime routine. These practices help calm the mind, reduce stress, and prepare your body for sleep.

· Limit Stimulants and Electronic Devices: Minimize the consumption of caffeine and avoid stimulating activities, such as intense exercise or screen time, close to bedtime.

The blue light emitted by electronic devices can interfere with your sleep quality, so it's best to limit their use before bed.

By integrating regular exercise, effective stress management techniques, and prioritizing quality sleep, you create a foundation for optimal well-being and support your kidney health. Experiment with different strategies to find what works best for you, and remember to consult with your healthcare professional for personalized recommendations based on your specific needs and health condition.

COLLABORATING WITH HEALTHCARE PROFESSIONALS AND SUPPORT NETWORKS

Managing kidney disease requires a comprehensive approach that involves collaborating with healthcare professionals and leveraging support networks. Here's a look at how these collaborations can enhance your kidney health journey:

Healthcare Professionals:

Nephrologist: Your nephrologist is a key member of your healthcare team who specializes in kidney care. They play a crucial role in diagnosing and monitoring your kidney condition, developing treatment plans, and providing guidance on managing kidney disease. Regular follow-up appointments with your nephrologist allow for ongoing assessment of your kidney function and adjustments to your treatment plan as needed.

Renal Dietitian: A renal dietitian is a specialized healthcare professional with expertise in kidney nutrition. Working closely with a renal dietitian can help you navigate the complexities of dietary management for kidney disease. They can provide personalized guidance on nutrient requirements, meal planning, and adapting your diet to suit your individual needs and preferences. Collaborating with a renal dietitian ensures that you receive tailored dietary recommendations to support your kidney health.

Other Specialists: Depending on your specific health needs, your healthcare team may include other specialists such as cardiologists, endocrinologists, or mental health professionals. Collaborating with these experts allows for a holistic approach to managing your overall health and addressing any co-existing conditions or complications related to kidney disease.

Support Networks:

Support Groups: Joining a support group for individuals with kidney disease can provide invaluable emotional support, practical tips, and a sense of community. Engaging with others who share similar experiences can help you feel understood, reduce feelings of isolation, and provide insights into coping strategies. Support groups may be available through local hospitals, community organizations, or online platforms.

Online Communities: Utilize online platforms and social media groups dedicated to kidney health. These communities can connect you with individuals worldwide who are navigating similar journeys. Share your experiences, seek advice, and contribute to discussions to benefit from a diverse range of perspectives and knowledge.

Family and Friends: Your loved ones play a crucial role in providing emotional support throughout your kidney health journey. Communicate openly with your family and friends about your condition, your needs, and how they can support you. Their understanding, encouragement, and involvement can make a significant difference in your overall well-being.

Remember, effective collaboration with healthcare professionals and active engagement with support networks can provide valuable insights, guidance, and emotional support as you navigate kidney disease. Regular communication with your healthcare team ensures that you stay informed about your condition, receive appropriate medical interventions, and make informed decisions about your treatment. Embrace the support available to you, and don't hesitate to seek assistance when needed.

YOUR KIDNEY HEALTH JOURNEY: STAYING ON TRACK

Maintaining a kidney-healthy lifestyle is a lifelong commitment that requires long-term adherence, motivation, and the ability to overcome challenges. In this chapter, we will delve into strategies to help you stay on track, overcome obstacles, and celebrate successes as you sustain kidney health for life.

LONG-TERM ADHERENCE AND MOTIVATION FOR A KIDNEY-HEALTHY LIFESTYLE

Maintaining a kidney-healthy lifestyle requires long-term adherence and consistent motivation. Here's a look at strategies to help you stay committed and motivated on your kidney health journey:

Reflect on Your Why: Regularly remind yourself of the reasons why you are committed to maintaining kidney health. Consider the impact it has on your overall well-being, quality of life, and the potential for slowing the progression of kidney disease. Connecting with your underlying motivations strengthens your resolve and reinforces your commitment to making kidney-healthy choices.

Set Realistic and Achievable Goals: Break down your long-term goals into smaller, manageable steps. Setting realistic and achievable goals allows you to celebrate milestones along the way, providing a sense of accomplishment and motivation. Focus on gradual progress rather than striving for perfection, recognizing that every positive choice you make contributes to your overall kidney health.

Stay Educated and Informed: Continuously seek knowledge about kidney health, nutrition, and advancements in treatment options. Stay informed about the latest research and recommendations from reputable sources. This empowers you to make informed decisions, adapt your lifestyle as needed, and reinforce your commitment to maintaining kidney health.

Embrace a Holistic Approach: Recognize that maintaining kidney health is not just about dietary choices but also involves other lifestyle factors. Embrace a holistic approach that incorporates regular physical activity, stress management techniques, adequate sleep, and emotional well-being. Addressing these aspects of your life supports overall health and can enhance your motivation to stay on track.

Find Support and Accountability: Surround yourself with a supportive network of family, friends, and healthcare professionals who understand your goals and provide encouragement. Share your journey with them and communicate your needs. Engaging in support groups or online communities of individuals with kidney disease can also provide valuable insights, encouragement, and accountability.

Celebrate Your Progress: Take time to acknowledge and celebrate your achievements along the way. Celebrating milestones, no matter how small, reinforces positive behavior and boosts motivation. Whether it's reaching a target blood pressure level, achieving weight loss goals, or consistently following your prescribed medication and dietary regimen, these accomplishments deserve recognition.

Practice Self-Care: Prioritize self-care activities that promote physical, mental, and emotional well-being. This may include engaging in relaxation techniques, practicing mindfulness or meditation, pursuing hobbies and interests, and engaging in activities that bring you joy and fulfillment. Nurturing yourself holistically enhances your overall motivation and supports your commitment to a kidney-healthy lifestyle.

Remember that maintaining long-term adherence and motivation requires dedication, patience, and self-compassion. Embrace the journey as an ongoing process of self-care and personal growth.

OVERCOMING CHALLENGES AND EMBRACING HEALTHY HABITS

Maintaining healthy habits for kidney health is an empowering journey, and overcoming challenges along the way only makes your success sweeter. Here are some uplifting insights to help you overcome obstacles and wholeheartedly embrace your healthy habits:

Embrace the Power of Possibility: Recognize that challenges are opportunities for growth and transformation. Each hurdle you face is a chance to discover your inner strength, resilience, and determination. Believe in yourself and trust that you have the capacity to overcome any challenge that comes your way.

Surround Yourself with Support: Build a network of uplifting individuals who believe in your ability to achieve your kidney health goals. Share your journey with loved ones, friends, or support groups who provide encouragement, understanding, and inspiration. Their unwavering support will bolster your motivation and remind you of your incredible capabilities.

Adapt and Thrive: Life is dynamic, and challenges may arise unexpectedly. Embrace the mindset of adaptability and flexibility. When faced with hurdles, take a deep breath and seek creative solutions. Embracing the ability to adapt allows you to find alternative paths, modify your strategies, and maintain your healthy habits with grace and resilience.

Celebrate Progress, Big and Small: Every step forward is a reason to celebrate. Acknowledge and appreciate the progress you make on your kidney health journey, no matter how small. Celebrate the milestones you reach, whether it's consistently incorporating more kidney-friendly foods into your meals, staying active with regular exercise, or mastering stress management techniques. Each achievement is a testament to your unwavering commitment and deserves recognition.

Practice Gratitude: Cultivate an attitude of gratitude for your journey. Reflect on the positive changes and improvements you have experienced along the way. Express gratitude for your body's resilience, the support you receive, and the opportunities to prioritize your kidney health. Embracing gratitude amplifies your motivation and nurtures a positive mindset that fuels your ongoing success.

Embody Self-Compassion: Be gentle and understanding with yourself during challenging times. Remember that setbacks are temporary and part of the growth process. Offer yourself love, compassion, and forgiveness if you veer off track or encounter obstacles. Treat yourself with the same kindness and understanding you would extend to a loved one, and use setbacks as opportunities to learn and grow stronger.

Believe in the Power of Your Choices: Remind yourself that each healthy choice you make is a powerful step towards nurturing your kidney health and overall well-being. Trust in the positive impact of your decisions and the cumulative effect they have on your journey. Your dedication and commitment are transforming your life, enhancing your vitality, and setting the stage for long-lasting wellness.

Embrace the Journey: Embrace your kidney health journey as a transformative and empowering experience. View challenges as opportunities for personal growth, self-discovery, and empowerment. With every hurdle you overcome, you become stronger, wiser, and more resilient. Embrace the beauty of the process and celebrate the amazing person you are becoming.

CELEBRATING SUCCESSES AND EMBRACING LIFELONG KIDNEY HEALTH

Your kidney health journey is a remarkable achievement, and celebrating your successes along the way is essential for maintaining long-term motivation and sustaining kidney health for life.

Recognize Your Progress: Take a moment to reflect on how far you have come on your kidney health journey. Celebrate the positive changes you have made, both big and small. Whether it's achieving your target blood pressure, improving lab results, or successfully incorporating kidney-friendly habits into your daily life, acknowledge the progress you have made and the positive impact it has had on your well-being.

Celebrate Milestones: Set specific milestones and goals to celebrate along your kidney health journey. These milestones can be anything that symbolizes your progress and achievements, such as sticking to your dietary plan for a certain period, consistently engaging in physical activity, or reaching a specific target in your treatment plan. Celebrate each milestone with a meaningful reward or acknowledgment that resonates with you.

Share Your Success: Share your successes with your support network. Let your loved ones, friends, or healthcare team know about your accomplishments. Sharing your journey and celebrating your successes not only boosts your own motivation but also inspires and encourages others who may be facing similar challenges. Your triumphs can create a ripple effect of positivity and motivation within your community.

Cultivate a Positive Mindset: Maintain a positive and optimistic mindset throughout your kidney health journey. Focus on the progress you have made rather than dwelling on setbacks or challenges. Celebrate your ability to overcome obstacles and use them as learning experiences that contribute to your growth and resilience. Embrace a mindset of gratitude, affirmations, and self-belief to sustain your motivation and drive.

Practice Self-Care and Reward Yourself: Incorporate self-care activities into your routine as a way to celebrate your commitment to kidney health. Engage in activities that bring you joy, relaxation, and rejuvenation. It could be taking a relaxing bath, enjoying a favorite hobby, spending quality time with loved ones, or treating yourself to something special that aligns with your kidney-healthy lifestyle. These acts of self-care not only celebrate your achievements but also reinforce the importance of prioritizing your well-being.

Embrace Lifelong Commitment: Recognize that kidney health is a lifelong journey, and sustaining your progress requires continued commitment and dedication. Celebrate the fact that you have embarked on a path of lifelong well-being and prioritize your kidney health as an integral part of your overall lifestyle. Embrace the opportunity to continue learning, growing, and adapting your habits to support long-term kidney health.

Stay Connected and Engaged: Stay connected with your healthcare team and support networks even after reaching specific milestones. Regularly check in with your healthcare professionals, attend follow-up appointments, and participate in support groups or online communities focused on kidney health. Engaging in ongoing discussions and sharing experiences with others who understand the challenges and triumphs can provide ongoing inspiration and support.

AVOIDING COMMON DIET MISTAKES

Navigating a kidney-friendly diet can be challenging, and it's natural to make mistakes along the way. In this chapter, we'll delve deeper into some common diet mistakes kidney patients make and offer detailed guidance on how to avoid them. Our goal is to provide you with the knowledge and tools to make informed choices about your diet, better manage your kidney disease, and improve your overall health.

One common mistake is over-restricting and unnecessarily eliminating foods. It's understandable to feel overwhelmed by dietary restrictions, but eliminating foods that are not necessarily harmful can result in an unbalanced and nutritionally inadequate diet. Instead of cutting out entire food groups, focus on portion control and moderation. Work closely with a renal dietitian to create a personalized meal plan that meets your nutritional needs while accommodating your taste preferences.

Another mistake is failing to individualize your diet based on your health and lab results. Kidney disease affects individuals differently, and **a one-size-fits-all approach to diet is not optimal**. It's crucial to tailor your diet to your specific health needs and lab results. Factors such as your stage of kidney disease, other medical conditions, and nutrient levels should all be taken into consideration. Collaborating with your healthcare team and renal dietitian will help you develop a customized dietary strategy that supports your unique situation.

A common error is relying too heavily on supplements instead of whole foods. While supplements can be beneficial in certain cases, they should not replace a balanced diet. Over-reliance on supplements can lead to nutrient imbalances and other health issues. Focus on obtaining nutrients from a variety of whole foods, and use supplements only as directed by your healthcare team. Remember, supplements should complement, not substitute, a well-rounded diet.

It's important to be cautious about following diet advice from random strangers on social media sites. While social media can offer valuable information and support, it's crucial to verify the credibility of the sources. Some individuals may share misleading or even harmful recommendations based on their own experiences or beliefs. Always consult your healthcare team and renal dietitian before making significant changes to your diet, and approach online advice with skepticism if it seems too good to be true or contradicts professional guidance.

Not reading food labels is another mistake that can negatively impact your kidney health. Many packaged foods contain hidden additives, preservatives, and excess sodium, which can be detrimental to your kidneys. Make it a habit to carefully read food labels and choose products with fewer ingredients and less processed components. Prioritize consuming real, whole foods that support your nutritional needs and overall health.

Additionally, not experimenting with food combinations,

cooking methods, and seasonings can lead to dietary monotony. Eating the same foods and dishes repeatedly can be tiresome and make it challenging to stick to a kidney-friendly diet. To add variety and excitement to your meals, be open to trying new food combinations, exploring different cooking methods, and experimenting with a range of seasonings and spices. Get creative in the kitchen, explore new recipes, and discover flavors that align with your dietary restrictions.

Managing your diet as a kidney patient can be complex, but it's an essential aspect of managing your kidney disease. By avoiding these common mistakes and working closely with your healthcare team, you can develop a personalized dietary strategy that supports your overall health and well-being. Remember, every journey has its challenges, but with patience, persistence, and a caring support system, you can confidently navigate your kidney-friendly diet.

FOODS WITH MAGICAL POWERS: DEBUNKING KIDNEY DIET FADS

Welcome to the whimsical world of "Foods with Magical Powers," where the internet is brimming with all sorts of kidney diet fads promising extraordinary benefits for your kidney health. In this chapter, we'll take a lighthearted journey through the land of exaggerated claims and dubious remedies promoted by the infamous "Dr. Facebook" and "Nurse TikTok." While these magical foods may captivate our attention with their enchanting promises, it's essential to approach them with a healthy dose of skepticism. Remember, when it comes to kidney health, scientific evidence and the guidance of healthcare professionals are your most reliable compass. So, let's embark on this amusing adventure as we explore the truth behind the hype and separate fact from fiction.

Magical Food #1: Apple Cider Vinegar:

One of the most frequently touted magical elixirs is apple cider vinegar (ACV). Advocates claim it can cure all ailments, including kidney disease. However, it's important to note that there is no scientific evidence supporting these grandiose claims. In fact, drinking ACV straight can be harmful to your dental health. The acidic nature of ACV can erode tooth enamel, leading to dental problems. While ACV can add a tangy flavor to salad dressings and other dishes, it should be consumed in moderation as part of a well-balanced diet, rather than relying on it as a cure-all for kidney health.

Magical Food #2: Special Waters:

The market is flooded with an array of "special waters" that claim to possess extraordinary properties for kidney health. However, the truth is that these waters offer little, if any, significant benefits beyond regular drinking water. The key to kidney health lies in proper hydration, and that can be achieved by simply drinking plain, refreshing water. Don't let the marketing trick you into spending a fortune on water with dubious claims. Stick to staying hydrated with plain, economical water, which is beneficial for your overall well-being.

Magical Food #3: Turmeric:

Turmeric, a vibrant golden spice, has gained popularity for its potential anti-inflammatory properties. While it is true that turmeric contains a compound called curcumin, which has shown promising effects in studies, its direct impact on kidney health remains inconclusive. While it can be enjoyed as a flavorful addition to dishes, it is important to understand that it is not a magical cure for kidney disease.

Magical Food #4: Celery Juice:

Celery juice has become a wellness trend, touted for its detoxifying and healing properties. However, it is essential to approach these claims with caution. While celery is a hydrating and nutritious vegetable, there is limited scientific evidence to support the specific benefits of drinking celery juice for kidney health. As part of a balanced diet, celery can contribute to overall well-being, but it should not be regarded as a magical potion for kidney rejuvenation.

Magical Food #5: Dandelion Tea:

Dandelion tea, made from the leaves and roots of the dandelion plant, has been praised for its potential diuretic properties and liver support. While it may offer some benefits, such as promoting fluid balance, there is no concrete evidence to support its direct impact on kidney health. As with any herbal tea, it is important to consume it in moderation and consider individual factors such as medication interactions or existing health conditions.

Magical Food #6: St. John's Wort:

St. John's Wort is an herb commonly used as a natural remedy for mild depression and anxiety. However, its effects on kidney health are not well-studied, and its use should be approached with caution. St. John's Wort may interact with certain medications, including those commonly prescribed to manage kidney disease. It is crucial to consult with your healthcare team before using this herb to ensure its safety and appropriateness for your specific situation.

Magical Food #7: Ephedra:

Ephedra, also known as ma huang, is a plant-derived substance that has been historically used for weight loss and athletic performance. However, it has been associated with serious health risks, including elevated blood pressure, heart problems, and kidney damage. Due to its potential for harm, ephedra has been banned in many countries, including the United States. It is essential to avoid products containing ephedra and prioritize your kidney health by focusing on evidence-based dietary strategies.

Remember that true progress in managing kidney disease comes from evidence-based practices, personalized nutrition plans, and the guidance of healthcare professionals. While some of these magical foods may be enjoyed in reasonable portions for flavor and variety, it's crucial to be skeptical of claims that promise extraordinary results without scientific backing. Embrace a balanced, well-rounded kidney diet rooted in sound nutrition principles, and you'll be on your way to supporting your kidney health in a practical and realistic way. Remember, it's the collective effort of a nutritious diet, lifestyle modifications, and professional guidance that truly unlocks the potential for thriving with kidney disease.

FREQUENTLY ASKED QUESTIONS: FOOD AND KIDNEY DISEASE

In this chapter, we will address common questions and concerns about specific foods and explore the impact of various foods on kidney health. It is important to note that the answers provided in this book are generalizations, and it is crucial to consult with your healthcare team or dietitian to get individualized answers that are unique to your own health and specific needs. By providing detailed insights, we aim to dispel misconceptions and provide clarity on how different foods can affect kidney health. Let's delve into the following:

ADDRESSING COMMON QUESTIONS AND CONCERNS ABOUT SPECIFIC FOODS

Are potatoes safe for kidney health?

- Potatoes can be a part of a kidney-healthy diet when prepared in the right way. It is important to limit the portion size and choose healthier cooking methods like baking or boiling instead of frying. Additionally, removing the skin can help reduce potassium content. Consulting with your healthcare team or dietitian will provide personalized guidance on incorporating potatoes into your specific meal plan.

Can I consume dairy products?

- Dairy products can be consumed in moderation as part of a kidney-healthy diet. However, it is important to choose lower phosphorus options like low-fat or skim milk, yogurt, or cheese. Your healthcare team or dietitian can help determine the appropriate portion sizes and guide you based on your individual needs and any underlying conditions.

What about chocolate and other sweets?

- Sweets and chocolates can be enjoyed in moderation as occasional treats. However, it is important to choose options with lower phosphorus and potassium content. Dark chocolate with a higher cocoa percentage can be a better choice due to its lower sugar content. Your healthcare team or dietitian can provide guidance on portion control and frequency based on your specific dietary requirements.

Is coffee or tea harmful?

- In general, moderate coffee and tea consumption is considered safe for most individuals with kidney disease. However, it is important to be mindful of caffeine intake, as excessive amounts can potentially increase blood pressure. In addition, be mindful of any additives which may contain sugar, phosphorus, or "empty" calories. If you have any specific concerns or recommendations regarding coffee or tea consumption, it is best to consult with your healthcare team or dietitian.

Should I avoid nuts and seeds?

- Nuts and seeds can be a part of a kidney-healthy diet, as they provide essential nutrients and healthy fats. However, they can be high in phosphorus, so it is important to choose lower phosphorus options and limit portion sizes. Soaking or roasting them can help reduce phosphorus content. Your healthcare team or dietitian can guide you on the appropriate amounts and types of nuts and seeds to include in your diet.

Can I enjoy spicy foods?

- Spicy foods can generally be consumed in moderation as part of a kidney-healthy diet. However, some individuals may find that spicy foods can cause digestive discomfort or heartburn. If you have any specific concerns or sensitivities, it is best to consult with your healthcare team or dietitian to determine the appropriate level of spiciness for your individual needs.

What are the considerations with regard to canned and processed foods?

- Canned and processed foods often contain higher amounts of sodium and phosphorus, so it is important to read labels carefully and choose low-sodium or phosphorus-modified options whenever possible. Rinsing canned foods can also help reduce sodium content. Fresh or homemade alternatives are generally encouraged, as they provide more control over ingredients and can be tailored to meet your specific dietary needs.

Can I use oil in my recipes?

- While it is generally recommended to limit oil intake for overall health, using small amounts of healthy oils, such as olive oil or avocado oil, can be part of a kidney-healthy diet. These oils provide beneficial monounsaturated fats. However, it is important to moderate the amount of oil used in cooking and opt for healthier cooking methods like sautéing or baking instead of deep-frying. Your healthcare team or dietitian can provide specific recommendations based on your individual needs.

Is one type of water better than another?

- When it comes to hydration, staying adequately hydrated

is more important than the specific type of water consumed. Drinking plain water is generally the best choice for maintaining kidney health. Bottled or filtered water can be a convenient option to avoid excessive sodium or minerals. However, there is no one-size-fits-all answer, and it is essential to consider individual circumstances. Consulting with your healthcare team or dietitian can help determine the most suitable type of water for your specific needs.

Can I eat bread?

- Bread can be included in a kidney-healthy diet, but it is important to choose the right type and moderate portion sizes. Opt for whole grain or whole wheat bread instead of refined white bread to benefit from its higher fiber content. Additionally, be mindful of sodium content and choose lower-sodium options when available. Your healthcare team or dietitian can guide you on the appropriate amount and type of bread to include in your diet.

Can I eat fish?

- Fish can be a valuable source of lean protein and healthy fats in a kidney-healthy diet. Certain types of fish, such as salmon, tuna, or mackerel, are rich in omega-3 fatty acids, which have anti-inflammatory properties and may be beneficial for kidney health. However, it is important to be mindful of phosphorus and potassium content. Opt for fresh or frozen fish and avoid breaded or processed varieties. Your healthcare team or dietitian can provide specific recommendations on portion sizes and frequency of fish consumption based on your individual needs.

Is Apple Cider Vinegar good for kidneys?

- There is no strong scientific evidence to suggest that apple cider vinegar specifically benefits kidney health. While some studies suggest that it may have potential health benefits, it is important to consult with your healthcare team or dietitian before incorporating apple cider vinegar into your kidney-healthy diet. They can provide guidance based on your individual health condition and any underlying concerns.

You keep stressing talking to my healthcare team - why doesn't one answer work for everyone?

· It is important to emphasize the importance of consulting with your healthcare team because kidney disease management is highly individualized. Each person's health condition, lab results, underlying conditions, and lifestyle factors can vary significantly. A renal diet is not a one-size-fits-all approach, as the nutritional needs of individuals with kidney disease can differ greatly. Additionally, the impact of dietary choices on kidney health can vary among individuals. While general guidelines for a kidney-healthy diet exist, such as managing sodium, phosphorus, and potassium intake, the specific limits and recommendations may differ based on individual circumstances. Working with your healthcare team ensures that your dietary plan aligns with your specific needs and goals, promoting optimal kidney health and overall wellness.

EXPLORING THE IMPACT OF VARIOUS FOODS ON KIDNEY HEALTH

The role of fruits and vegetables in kidney health:

· Fruits and vegetables are rich in essential nutrients, antioxidants, and fiber, making them vital components of a kidney-healthy diet. They provide a wide range of vitamins, minerals, and phytochemicals that support overall health and help reduce the risk of chronic diseases. Including a variety of colorful fruits and vegetables in your diet can provide valuable nutrients while being mindful of potassium and phosphorus content. Working with your healthcare team or dietitian can help you identify suitable options based on your individual needs.

Understanding protein sources and their impact on kidney function:

- Protein is an essential nutrient for maintaining muscle mass and supporting overall health. However, excessive protein intake can strain the kidneys, especially in individuals with kidney disease. It is important to choose high-quality protein sources, such as lean meats, poultry, fish, eggs, dairy products, and plant-based proteins like legumes, tofu, and tempeh. Balancing protein intake with your healthcare team or dietitian's guidance helps ensure you meet your nutritional needs while minimizing kidney stress.

The importance of managing sodium and phosphorus intake:

- Sodium and phosphorus are two minerals that require careful management in a kidney-healthy diet. High sodium intake can contribute to fluid retention and increased blood pressure, while excessive phosphorus intake can disrupt mineral balance and lead to complications. Monitoring and limiting sodium and phosphorus intake by choosing low-sodium alternatives, reducing processed and fast foods, and controlling portion sizes can help maintain kidney health and prevent complications associated with kidney disease.

Balancing carbohydrates and sugars in the diet:

- Carbohydrates are an important source of energy, but it is essential to choose them wisely and balance their intake. Opting for complex carbohydrates, such as whole grains, legumes, and vegetables, provides fiber and nutrients while promoting stable blood sugar levels. It is also important to be mindful of added sugars, as excessive sugar intake can contribute to weight gain and increased risk of diabetes, which can further impact kidney health. Moderation and focusing on whole food sources of carbohydrates are key.

Exploring the benefits of healthy fats and oils:

- Healthy fats and oils, such as monounsaturated and polyunsaturated fats, play a crucial role in supporting overall health, including kidney health. Sources like avocados, nuts, seeds, and olive oil provide essential fatty acids and help reduce inflammation. It is important to incorporate these healthy fats in moderation while being mindful of overall calorie intake, as excessive fat consumption can contribute to weight gain.

The impact of different cooking methods on nutrient content:

- The way we cook our food can affect the nutrient content. Certain cooking methods, such as boiling and steaming, are better for preserving nutrients compared to deep-frying or prolonged high-heat cooking. Opting for gentler cooking methods can help retain the nutritional value of foods, ensuring you receive the maximum benefits from your meals.

EVIDENCE-BASED INSIGHTS TO DISPEL MYTHS AND MISCONCEPTIONS

Let's now address common myths and misconceptions surrounding food and kidney health. It is important to rely on scientific evidence and expert guidance to make informed decisions about your dietary choices. Let's explore some evidence-based insights that can help dispel these myths:

Myth: "A kidney-healthy diet means completely avoiding protein."

- Fact: While excessive protein intake can strain the kidneys, it is important to consume an adequate amount of high-quality protein to meet your nutritional needs. Working with your healthcare team or dietitian to determine the appropriate amount of protein for your individual condition is crucial. They can help you strike the right balance that supports kidney health without compromising your overall nutritional requirements.

Myth: "All fruits and vegetables are high in potassium and should be avoided."

- Fact: While some fruits and vegetables are indeed high in potassium, many others are lower in potassium content and can be safely included in a kidney-healthy diet. The key is to work with your healthcare team or dietitian to identify suitable options based on your specific potassium needs. They can guide you in selecting fruits and vegetables that are lower in potassium and suggest appropriate portion sizes to fit your dietary plan.

Myth: "A kidney-healthy diet is tasteless and boring."

- Fact: A kidney-healthy diet can be both nutritious and delicious. By exploring various herbs, spices, and low-sodium seasonings, you can enhance the flavors of your meals without compromising your kidney health. Additionally, experimenting with different cooking techniques, using fresh ingredients, and exploring new recipes can add excitement and variety to your meals while adhering to your dietary guidelines.

Myth: "I can rely on dietary supplements instead of a kidney-healthy diet."

- Fact: While certain supplements may have their place in managing specific nutrient deficiencies, they should not be seen as a substitute for a well-balanced kidney-healthy diet. Whole foods provide a wide range of nutrients, fiber, and other beneficial compounds that work synergistically to support your overall health. It is important to focus on obtaining nutrients from real food sources and consult with your healthcare team before considering any dietary supplements.

Myth: "A kidney-healthy diet means completely avoiding all salt."

- Fact: While reducing sodium intake is important for kidney health, it does not mean eliminating salt entirely. Sodium is present in many natural foods, and some amount of salt is necessary for proper bodily functions. The key is to limit excessive sodium intake from processed and packaged foods and instead opt for lower-sodium alternatives and seasonings.

Myth: "All herbal teas are safe for kidney health."

- Fact: While herbal teas can have various health benefits, certain herbal teas may contain compounds that can be harmful to the kidneys. It is essential to consult with your healthcare team or dietitian to determine which herbal teas are safe for you to consume, especially if you have underlying kidney conditions or take specific medications.

Myth: "I should avoid all dairy products in a kidney-healthy diet."

- Fact: Dairy products can be part of a kidney-healthy diet, as they are a good source of high-quality protein and essential nutrients like calcium and vitamin D. However, it is important to choose lower-fat or fat-free options and consume them in moderation based on your individual dietary plan.

Myth: "Eating too much protein can cure or reverse kidney disease."

- Fact: While a balanced intake of high-quality protein

is essential for overall health, it cannot cure or reverse kidney disease. Managing protein intake, along with other dietary and lifestyle modifications, can help slow the progression of kidney disease and maintain optimal kidney function.

Myth: "All herbal supplements are safe for kidney health."

- Fact: Herbal supplements may have potential interactions with medications or contain substances that can be harmful to the kidneys. It is important to consult with your healthcare team before taking any herbal supplements to ensure they are safe and appropriate for your specific kidney health needs.

Myth: "A kidney-healthy diet is only for people with advanced kidney disease."

- Fact: A kidney-healthy diet is beneficial for individuals at all stages of kidney disease, including those with early-stage kidney disease or at risk for developing kidney problems. Adopting a kidney-healthy lifestyle can help preserve kidney function, manage symptoms, and promote overall well-being.

Myth: "I can drink as much water as I want to flush out my kidneys."

- Fact: While adequate hydration is important for kidney health, excessive water intake can strain the kidneys, especially in individuals with compromised kidney function. It is essential to maintain a balance and follow your healthcare team's or dietitian's recommendations regarding fluid intake based on your individual needs.

Myth: "All processed foods are off-limits in a kidney-healthy diet."

- Fact: While processed foods are generally higher in sodium and additives, not all processed foods need to be completely avoided. It is important to read labels carefully, choose lower-sodium options, and focus on incorporating whole, unprocessed foods as the foundation of your diet.

Myth: "I can skip my medications if I follow a kidney-healthy diet."

- Fact: A kidney-healthy diet is a valuable addition to managing kidney disease but should never replace prescribed medications. Dietary modifications should be implemented in conjunction with medical treatments and under the guidance of your healthcare team.

Myth: "Kidney disease only affects older adults, so I don't need to worry about it."

- Fact: While the risk of kidney disease increases with age, it can affect individuals of any age, including children and young adults. It is essential to adopt a kidney-healthy lifestyle, including proper nutrition, at all stages of life to promote kidney health and prevent the progression of kidney disease.

RESOURCES

In your journey with kidney disease and navigating the kidney diet, it's important to recognize that there is a vast array of resources available to help you learn and understand more about your condition. Never stop seeking knowledge and exploring the wealth of information that can support you in making informed decisions about your health. From reputable websites and online platforms to specialized organizations and community support, these resources can provide valuable insights, practical tips, and the latest research on kidney disease and the kidney diet. By actively engaging with these resources, you empower yourself to take control of your health and well-being. Remember, knowledge is power, and the more you learn, the better equipped you are to thrive with kidney disease.

Dadvice TV Kidney Health Coach YouTube Channel

Dadvice TV is a beacon of hope in an otherwise murky sea of confusion and uncertainty. With unparalleled enthusiasm and positivity, James Fabin and industry professionals delve into a plethora of topics ranging from kidney disease symptoms to treatment options, and from dietary and lifestyle changes to savvy insights which enable those suffering from kidney disease to take informed decisions regarding their health and well-being. Dadvice TV's unwavering mission is to inspire and empower people with kidney disease to not only survive but thrive, by providing them with the tools and knowledge necessary to lead healthier and longer lives.

Plant-Powered Kidneys Website & Facebook Group

Plant-Powered Kidneys, Inc. was founded in 2018 by board-certified Renal Dietitian Jen Hernandez. PPK has since become one of the top leaders in providing safe and evidence-based renal nutrition information for kidney patients worldwide.

Jen has worked with kidney patients in every stage of CKD, including dialysis and transplant. It was when she worked in dialysis and became so sad with the new patients pouring into the clinics every week that she decided to get ahead of the problem.

With a deer-in-headlights look on their, her dialysis patients say, "I wish I made some changes to my diet before it came to this. I had no idea it could change so fast."

So Jen set out to create a space online that provided nutrition education to those that wanted to make that difference. To prevent kidney failure and protect their kidney health.

From free meal plans and recipes to CKD nutrition blog articles, Plant-Powered Kidneys provides evidence-based information.

Jen and Plant-Powered Kidneys have been featured in national publications, including Healthline, U.S. News, and The National Kidney Foundation. Jen has also received awards for her work in patient education.

For those ready to take renal nutrition into their own hands, PPK offers an online course that covers the pillars of renal nutrition. Over 1,000 students have taken the course and report less anxiety over their food, more meal options to support kidney health, and skyrocketed confidence in speaking with their healthcare team about their individual kidney health. In fact, 2 out of 3 students that have taken the course report improved labs, and 75% of students are very confident about cooking a kidney-healthy meal!

You can learn more and get the free resources Plant-Powered Kidneys has to offer by visiting their website.

Website: www.plantpoweredkidneys.com

Facebook: www.facebook.com/plantpoweredkidneys

Facebook group: www.facebook.com/groups/plantpoweredkidneys

Instagram: www.instagram.com/plantpoweredkidneys

YouTube: www.youtube.com/plantpoweredkidneys

Kidney Nutrition Institute

Kidney Nutrition Institute (KidneyNutritionInstitute.org) is a progressive renal nutrition practice that uses cutting-edge nutrition strategies to help people improve their kidney function. They take a functional-integrative approach that looks at root cause driving factors of kidney disease to help resolve the problem at its core, not just treat symptoms. Kidney Nutrition Institute has also been a pioneer especially in the world of polycystic kidney disease, helping pioneer the first plant-focused, kidney safe ketogenic dietary approach for PKD. This approach has been used successfully for other patients with metabolic abnormalities such as in the case of diabetes.

They provide a full range of services including meal planning, one-to-one personalized nutrition strategies, a resource database for patients who need ideas on what to eat and want to connect with other patients.

Outside of patient services, Kidney Nutrition Institute is a leader in the industry training renal dietitians on advanced therapies, developing educational resources, and consulting with organizations on research and implementation of best practice.

Cronometer Food Tracking App

Cronometer (http://go.DadviceTV.com/app) is a user-friendly food tracking app that can be a helpful tool in managing your kidney diet. It allows you to log your daily food intake, track nutrient values, and monitor your progress. With its extensive database, you can easily search for specific foods, including their nutrient composition, and make more informed choices. The app provides a convenient way to stay on top of your nutritional goals and ensure you're meeting your dietary needs.

USDA FoodData Central Database

The USDA FoodData Central is a comprehensive database that provides detailed information on the nutrient content of various foods. It offers an extensive collection of nutrient data, including minerals, vitamins, macronutrients, and more. This resource can help you make informed decisions when selecting foods and understanding their nutritional composition. It serves as a reliable source for accessing accurate and up-to-date nutrient information.

American Kidney Fund (AKF)

The American Kidney Fund is an invaluable resource for individuals seeking support and education about kidney disease. With a mission to fight kidney disease through direct financial assistance, education, and advocacy, the AKF offers a wealth of resources to empower and uplift those affected by kidney disease. Through their educational materials, online resources, and patient programs, the AKF provides valuable information on kidney health, treatment options, financial assistance programs, and support services. Their commitment to improving the lives of individuals with kidney disease is unwavering, and they serve as a beacon of hope and guidance for the kidney community. Whether you need help understanding your diagnosis, accessing financial aid, or finding support groups, the American Kidney Fund is dedicated to being a trusted ally on your kidney health journey. Website: https://www.kidneyfund.org/

National Kidney Foundation (NKF)

The National Kidney Foundation is a reputable organization dedicated to the awareness, prevention, and treatment of kidney disease. Their website provides a wide range of resources on kidney health, including information on the kidney diet. You can find educational materials, tips, recipes, and guidelines to support your dietary needs. Website: https://www.kidney.org/

American Association of Kidney Patients (AAKP)

The American Association of Kidney Patients is a patient-centered organization that offers resources and advocacy for individuals with kidney disease. Their website features educational content, including diet and nutrition information, to help you make informed decisions about your kidney health. They also provide opportunities for community engagement and support. Website: https://aakp.org/

Renal Dietitians Practice Group (RDPG)

The Renal Dietitians Practice Group is a specialized group within the Academy of Nutrition and Dietetics. They focus on providing evidence-based guidance and resources for renal dietitians and individuals with kidney disease. Visiting their website can give you access to resources, publications, and professional insights related to the kidney diet.

Kidney Kitchen

Kidney Kitchen is an online platform that offers kidney-friendly recipes and educational materials on nutrition for kidney health. They provide recipe ideas tailored to the needs of individuals with kidney disease, along with helpful tips for adapting meals to meet dietary restrictions. Exploring their website can inspire you to create delicious and nourishing meals while following your kidney diet. Website: https://kitchen.kidneyfund.org/

AKF Community Resource Finder

Using AKF's Community Resource Finder, powered by findhelp, users may enter their zip code so that they can be directed to a comprehensive list of local or regional programs broken into categories such as food, housing, care, and transit. Website: https://www.kidneyfund.org/community-resource-finder

Local Support Groups and Classes

Consider reaching out to local support groups or healthcare organizations that offer kidney disease support. They may provide educational classes, workshops, or group sessions focused on nutrition and the kidney diet. Connecting with others who share similar experiences can provide valuable support and guidance on your kidney health journey.

Renal Recipes (https://www.dadvicetv.com/recipes)

Discover a wide collection of free kidney-friendly renal recipes available online at the Dadvice TV website. These recipes are specifically designed to meet the dietary needs of individuals with kidney disease, providing delicious and nutritious meal options. You can find an extensive range of recipes offered by localized kidney groups and reputable kidney organizations from around the world. These recipes not only cater to the specific dietary restrictions of kidney disease but also emphasize flavor, variety, and culinary enjoyment. Exploring renal recipes allows you to expand your culinary repertoire and discover new ways to prepare kidney-friendly meals that are both nourishing and satisfying.

By utilizing these kidney diet resources, you can enhance your knowledge, access expert advice, and find support on your journey to better kidney health. Remember, always consult with your healthcare team and registered dietitian to ensure that the information you gather aligns with your specific needs and circumstances.

CONQUERING THE KIDNEY DIET: YOUR PATH TO SUCCESS

Congratulations! You have reached the final chapter of this book, and I want to take a moment to express my heartfelt admiration for your commitment to your health and well-being. Throughout this journey, we have explored the ins and outs of the kidney diet, and you have shown incredible determination and resilience.

I want you to know that your health matters deeply to me, and I genuinely care about your success in managing your kidney disease. Your decision to educate yourself, seek guidance, and make positive changes in your lifestyle is a testament to your strength and courage. I am here to remind you that you are not alone in this journey. You have a community of support standing beside you every step of the way.

As we wrap up this book, let's reflect on the key points that have empowered you to conquer the kidney diet. Remember, the impact of your dietary choices extends far beyond just your meals. By following the guidance of a renal dietitian, you have taken the first important step in personalizing your diet to suit your unique needs. Together, we have emphasized the significance of individualized nutrition and the transformative effects it can have on your kidney health.

I want to reassure you that the kidney diet is **not** about depriving yourself or living in fear of food. Instead, it's about finding a balance that supports your health and allows you to savor the joys of eating. With portion control and mindful choices, you can continue to enjoy a wide variety of delicious foods while safeguarding your kidney function. It's a journey of discovery, and you have already come so far.

While it may seem challenging at times, I want you to remember that every small step you take matters. It's not about achieving perfection but about making progress and consistently making choices that align with your goals. Be patient with yourself, and celebrate each milestone along the way. Your dedication to self-care and your commitment to your well-being are extraordinary.

I want to assure you that your efforts are not in vain. By managing your sodium intake, being mindful of phosphorus, embracing a balanced acid-base environment, and understanding the impact of various nutrients, you are proactively taking charge of your kidney health. It's not always an easy path, but I believe in your ability to overcome any obstacles that come your way.

As you navigate the kidney diet, remember that setbacks and challenges are a part of the journey. Don't be discouraged by temporary setbacks. Instead, view them as opportunities for growth and learning. Keep a positive mindset and focus on the progress you have made and the goals you have achieved. Believe in yourself, because I believe in you.

Finally, I want to express my deepest gratitude for allowing me to be a part of your kidney health journey. It has been an honor to share my knowledge and insights with you. Remember that I am here to support you, and I encourage you to reach out to me or seek support from your healthcare team whenever you need guidance or encouragement.

You are capable, resilient, and deserving of a vibrant and fulfilling life. With the knowledge, tools, and unwavering determination you have cultivated throughout this book, I have no doubt that you will conquer the kidney diet and thrive with kidney disease. Embrace the power within you, and let it guide you towards a future filled with health, happiness, and countless blessings.

Congratulations on embarking on this transformative journey. Your commitment to your health inspires me, and I am excited to witness the incredible impact you will have on your kidney health and overall well-being. Remember, you have the power to shape your own destiny and live a life that is not defined by kidney disease but rather by your unwavering spirit and determination. You've got this, and I am cheering you on every step of the way.

ABOUT THE AUTHOR

James Fabin

James Fabin is a devoted husband and loving father of two young children. Throughout his life, James has been an active participant in charitable endeavors, dedicating his time and resources to make a positive impact on the lives of others.

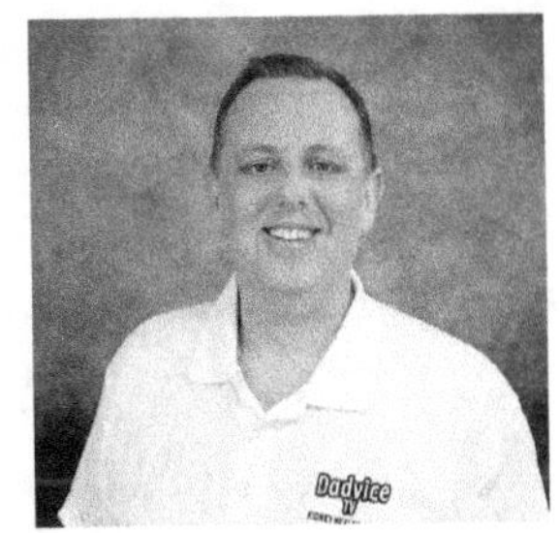

A passionate animal lover, James shares his home with two beloved dogs and volunteers with animal rescue groups, providing support and assistance to animals in need. His dedication to helping others, whether they have two legs or four, is evident in everything he does.

In his professional life, James works in the automotive industry, where he specializes in marketing. His expertise in this field has allowed him to connect with people from all walks of life and apply his skills to create meaningful and lasting relationships.

James's journey with chronic kidney disease has inspired him to share his knowledge and experience with others, providing valuable insights and practical advice through his writing. By combining his passion for helping others with his personal experiences, James hopes to empower those facing kidney disease to take control of their health and improve their quality of life.

Learn more about James and watch his ever-growing kidney video library at www.DadviceTV.com

BOOKS BY THIS AUTHOR

Conquering Kidney Disease: A Survivors Guide To Thriving With Ckd

Embark on a comprehensive journey through the world of kidney health with this definitive guide that intertwines scientific insight, practical advice, and a compassionate approach to managing kidney disease. This book is an invaluable resource for anyone who's grappling with the challenges of kidney disease, kidney failure, or simply wishes to understand the intricacies of kidney health better.

Discover the answers to your pressing questions about kidney disease, from its earliest stages to the potential of kidney failure. Learn the importance of early detection, understand how the disease progresses, and uncover the power of proactive management of your health. With detailed explanations made easy to understand, you'll gain a solid grasp of what chronic kidney disease (CKD) entails.

The book goes beyond just medical facts and delves into the everyday realities of living with kidney disease, offering practical advice on maintaining a kidney-friendly lifestyle. Central to this is the kidney diet. This book dispels the one-size-fits-all myth, emphasizing that a kidney diet should be as unique as you are. You'll learn about the significance of protein in your diet, the differences between animal and plant proteins, and how the right balance can help manage your condition.

Master the art of individualized diet planning with help from experts and real-life stories. This book encourages a collaborative care approach, urging the involvement of renal dietitians and healthcare teams in managing your kidney health. Explore different treatment options, including dialysis and kidney transplants, helping you make informed decisions about your health journey.

Armed with the latest research, personal anecdotes, and a wealth of practical tips, this book aims to inspire, educate, and empower you to take control of your kidney health. Whether you are a kidney patient yourself, a caretaker, or a health professional seeking to enhance your knowledge, this comprehensive guide presents a holistic view of kidney health. Navigate the landscape of kidney disease with confidence, armed with knowledge, and inspired to make the best choices for your unique journey.

www.ingramcontent.com/pod-product-compliance
Lightning Source LLC
Chambersburg PA
CBHW060036260726
48658CB00004B/1070